KU-484-299

Coping with Loss:
Helping patients and their families

Edited by

Colin Murray Parkes

Consultant Psychiatrist to St Christopher's Hospice, Sydenham, and St Joseph's Hospice, Hackney, London, UK

and

Andrew Markus

General Practitioner, Thame, Oxon and Emeritus Fellow, Green College, Oxford, UK

© BMJ Books 1998
BMJ Books is an imprint of the BMJ Publishing Group

All rights reserved. No part of this publication may be reproduced,
stored in a retrieval system, or transmitted, in any form or by any
means, electronic, mechanical, photocopying, recording and/or
otherwise, without the prior written permission of the publishers.

First published in 1998
by BMJ Books, BMA House, Tavistock Square,
London WC1H 9JR

British Library Cataloguing in Publication Data

A catalogue record for this book is available from the
British Library

ISBN 0-7279-1068-X

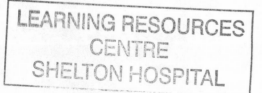
LEARNING RESOURCES
CENTRE
SHELTON HOSPITAL

Contents

Contributors

Glin Bennet, Former Consultant Senior Lecturer, Department of Mental Health, University of Bristol, and former Consultant Psychiatrist, United Bristol Healthcare NHS Trust, Bristol

Dora Black, Honorary Consultant Child and Adolescent Psychiatrist, Traumatic Stress Clinic, Charlotte Street, London, Great Ormond Street Hospital for Children, Tavistock Clinic, and Honorary Senior Lecturer in Psychiatry, Royal Free School of Medicine, London, and University College, London

Leonard Fagin, Consultant Psychiatrist and Honorary Senior Lecturer, South Forest Centre, Forest Healthcare Trust, and University College, London

Roy G Fitzgerald, Associate Clinical Professor of Psychiatry, Thomas Jefferson University, Philadelphia

Peter Maguire, Honorary Consultant Psychiatrist, Christie Hospital, Manchester, and Director, Cancer Research Campaign Psychological Medicine Group, Christie CRC Research Centre, University of Manchester, Manchester

Colin Murray Parkes, Consultant Psychiatrist to St Christopher's Hospice, Sydenham, and St Joseph's Hospice, Hackney

Brice Pitt, Former Professor, Psychiatry of Old Age, St Mary's Hospital Medical School, London

Robert S Weiss, Senior Fellow, Gerontology Institute, and Emeritus Professor, Department of Sociology, University of Massachusetts, Boston, Massachusetts

Foreword

"What does not kill me makes me stronger" said Rilke. "The way out is the way through" said Bishop Evered Lunt, our Spiritual Director as we planned St Christopher's Hospice. Loss can send us into a hectic round of activity, avoiding responsibility; it can lead to bitterness and inability to move forward, but encouragingly, even more often it may lead to growth if it is met head on.

It is not only as if the tragedy had never been, it is better than that; for the person has survived the loss, learnt and grown and emerges stronger. Hopefully, too, they will have a greater sympathy and understanding of others as they face their deprivations or bereavements. Many pioneering developments and charitable foundations have come from the "widened heart" and creative power which loss can generate. Sometimes, but certainly not always, this is seen as a religious calling to better the free and dangerous world in which bad things happen to good people.[1]

Loss takes many forms and few escape it in their lives. Here is a book coming from the life times' experience of people who have helped others along an often bleak journey. It will surely bring encouragement to those of us who wish to draw on their wisdom, and give us new confidence in the resilience of the human spirit and a greater readiness to stand by those of our fellows who are facing any kind of bereavement.

Dame Cicely Saunders, OM, DBE, FRCP
Chairman, St Christopher's Hospice, London.
May 1998.

1 Kushner, HS. *When Bad Things Happen to Good People*. Schocken Books, 1981.

1 Introduction

COLIN MURRAY PARKES

The ubiquity of loss

Doctors are acquainted with loss and grief. Not only do we witness it in the relatives of the dying and the bereaved, we come across it in many other situations. Our patients grieve for the numerous losses to which illness and accident give rise, and losses are a common cause of psychiatric disorders which may, in their turn, cause other losses. Doctors too are not immune from grief for the losses in our own lives, both those that all humans are heir to and those that arise because we care for and about our patients.

Some losses we inflict on our patients when we operate to remove a diseased organ or prescribe a drastic but necessary treatment. Often we do this deliberately for fear of something worse, but even treatments that are not normally damaging can sometimes cause unexpected loss and we are left to "pick up the pieces".

General practitioners frequently encounter loss. Thus, in a study by Clark of 200 consultations, 66 (33%) were thought to be psychological in origin.[1] Of these, 55 (83%) were identified as resulting from types of loss. In order of frequency the types of loss included separations from loved others, incapacitation, bereavement, migration, relocation, job losses, birth of a baby, retirement, and professional loss. These and some of the other types of loss which will be considered in this book are listed in box 1.1.

The damaging effects of loss

Loss can plague the lives of patients, relatives, and doctors. It contributes to depression, anxiety states, and many other psychiatric disorders. It can wreck marriages, ruin childhood,

1

<table>
<tr><td>

Box 1.1   Types of loss

Loss of relationships:

- by death
- by other cause (for example divorce)

Loss of body image
Loss of bodily functions

- Motor
- Sensory
- Cognitive

Loss of home/territory
Loss of roles and occupation
Loss of plans and hopes for the future
Loss of one's own life

</td></tr>
</table>

and drive people to drink. It causes many would-be doctors and nurses to give up medicine and can undermine the work satisfaction of those who remain. It is even a cause of death, contributing to mortality from heart disease, suicide, and other causes (Parkes reviews this literature[2]). Among the life events which Paykel found to be associated with clinical depression and with suicide attempts the commonest were "exits" and "undesirable".[3] Clegg found that a third of 71 people admitted to a psychiatric unit for elderly patients had suffered one or more recent bereavements.[4]

Despite this, there is also evidence that handled right losses can foster maturity and personal growth. Certainly there is no reason to believe that the effects of losses are always and necessarily harmful. The consequences of loss considered in this volume are listed in box 1.2.

Lack of recognition of the importance of loss

So distressing and far reaching are the consequences of loss that we might expect the topic to occupy a large place in the training of doctors and other providers of health care. But this is not the case. Until recent years grief was not even mentioned in textbooks

---

Box 1.2   Effects of loss

Psychological

- Grief and its complications
- Depression (with or without suicide risk)
- Anxiety states and panic disorders
- Substance abuse
- Other psychiatric disorders
- Increased maturity

Physical

- Autonomic, immune, and endocrine reactions
- Psychosomatic disorders
- Increased mortality

---

of psychiatry, and we have to go back to Richard Burton's *Anatomy of Melancholy*, published in 1621,[5] to find that loss was once accorded an important place in medicine. Burton refers to loss or sorrow as, "The epitome, symptome and chief cause of melancholie", and it was accepted that a "broken heart" could indeed be a cause of death from Biblical times to the 19th century.

Why should it be that a topic that is so central in importance receives so little attention today? One answer may be the assumption that loss is irreversible and untreatable; there is nothing we can do about it, and the best way of dealing with it is to ignore it. This attitude may help us to live with the painful fact that, despite all the advances of modern science, all our patients still die and before they die many will suffer lasting losses in their lives. Sadly, it also means that, just when they need us most, our patients and their grieving relatives often find that we back away. Perhaps we feel helpless because we do not know how to help, perhaps the whole topic depresses us (for we are all mortal), maybe we feel guilty of failing to cure, or we may just be too busy to give the care that is needed. For any or all of these reasons we attempt to distance ourselves from their grief. If we fail in this attempt we are likely to find

3

that our own peace of mind is disturbed. We may even fear that our ability to help others will be impaired if we do not keep a strict rein on our feelings. We learn the hard way to be hard or we pack up and clear out of medicine.

Recent approaches to loss and stress

This pessimistic view was challenged in 1944 by the publication of an important study by Lindemann of bereaved survivors of a night club fire.[6] Lindemann provided doctors with a way of thinking about and "treating" grief in much the same way as we think about and treat illness. At the same time he recognised it as a "normal" process which might go wrong, and he saw our function as restorative. In this one paper he confronted us with a problem and suggested a solution. His work sowed the seeds of our current understanding of the psychology of bereavement and led to the development of services for the bereaved.

Bereavement by death is, of course, only one of the many types of loss that come to medical attention, and Lindemann's ideas were soon applied to a wide range of other life crises. This in turn gave rise to "crisis intervention services" and fuelled interest in the emerging specialties of preventive psychiatry and community mental health.

A little known paper published in 1963 by Aldrich, *The Dying Patient's Grief*, extended this understanding to the griefs of the dying[7] and was taken up and developed by one of his trainee psychiatrists, Elizabeth Kubler Ross, whose book *On Death and Dying* proved seminal.[8] Suddenly we had something to offer "the hopeless case". Her work coincided with and provided a psychological dimension to the work on pain control and "holistic" care for the dying which was being developed by Cicely Saunders and other pioneers of the hospice movement.

More recently the improvements in care that were spearheaded in the hospices have extended to other settings and given rise to a new discipline—palliative medicine. Home care services have bridged the gap between hospice and home care for dying patients, and general practitioners have been taking a central role, not only in caring for dying patients and their families but also in supporting people through the many other losses which bring them into medical care. In 1989 Markus *et al* broke new ground by describing a model for mental health care by the primary care team which, instead of focusing on the treatment of mental illnesses, described the ways in which they can be prevented by recognising the various losses that people face at each stage of life and providing appropriate care.[9]

In parallel with the research into bereavement was research into the physiology and psychology of other noxious life events contained within the broad rubric of "stress".

Knowledge of the endocrinology, neurophysiology, and immunology of stress have all grown exponentially during this century and have helped to provide a frame of reference for our thinking about mind-body relations and, with the advent of stress psychology, a basis for various types of stress reduction. In 1960 the "crisis theory" of Parad and Caplan extended the concept of stress to include the social systems of family, workplace, and community but did little to draw together the "stress" and "loss" frames of reference.[10] A proper integration of these twin topics of study is only now coming about.

The taboos on death and bereavement have been broken, and a sexologist was recently heard to comment that, whereas a few years ago lectures to medical students on "sex" were always well attended it is now necessary to put the word "death" in the title if you want to get a large audience. This wave of curiosity and enthusiasm has created further problems. In the United States the interest in preventive psychiatry, which coincided with the provision of federal funds for the prevention of mental ill health in the 1960s, was followed by disillusionment when both the scientific justification and the funds failed to match the hopes of its proponents.

The pendulum swings back and forth, and it is not unreasonable to expect that the end result will be a gradual change in our attitudes and ways of working which takes account of well founded advances in scientific knowledge in this specialty and enables those aspects of service that are firmly based to be developed. All of this takes time, and we are still a long way from general acceptance of a systematic theory and research base. We should not be surprised if those who study the specialty sometimes adopt different viewpoints. In fact, there is no one way that is "right", humans are sufficiently complex for us to see them from more than one perspective.

This variation is reflected in the chapters in this book, which are written by eight authorities each from his or her own point of view. The editor has far too much respect for his coauthors to attempt to impose a single theoretical or practical model on them. Indeed, it is this very variety that adds depth and interest. Even so there are core concepts that link each chapter and go some way to explain the repeated finding that there is much that members of the caring professions can do to help people through the losses that so often become turning points in their lives. These are summarised in the final chapter.

The twin processes of grief and change

Two main processes are set in train by major losses: grief and the psychological and social changes which follow it. *Grief* is the normal reaction to a loss and is the means by which people begin to accept the reality of an event which will change their lives. The term *psychosocial transition* covers the complex process of learning which then takes place. The married person must learn to be a widow or widower, the intact person must discover what it means to be an amputee, the blind person must learn how to cope without sight. These are all part of the process of rehabilitation which must follow any major life change.[11]

In this book we shall examine how people experience the transitions caused by accident and illness, what happens inside the head of a person who goes blind, loses a limb, loses a spouse, or realises that he or she doesn't have long to live. This exercise will take us beyond the answer to the question, "What is it like to be blind, an amputee, a widow, or dying?" to the more important question, "How do people change from being sighted, two legged, a wife, or a person with a future into whatever it is that they become when they are not one of these things?"

The question is important for two very different types of reason. One is that as care givers we need to understand how illness and accident affect our patients and their families if we are to help them through these transitions. The other is a more personal reason. Sooner or later each of us will have to make one or other of these transitions for ourselves. We too will become patients or bereaved and will experience the fears and griefs of unwanted change in our lives; it is not unreasonable to hope that we shall find ourselves better prepared for these changes if we have anticipated them.

The anticipation of loss

This last consideration is, of course, quite crucial. We don't "look forward" to the things we don't look forward to. There is not much point in anticipating misery unless you can do something about it. We condemn John Donne, who used to sleep in a coffin to get used to the idea of being dead, and we may find people who work in hospices rather creepy (unless we are one of those people in which case, of course, we find them quite normal).

In fact there is a great deal of evidence, which will be reviewed, that *the anticipation of possible or probable change in our lives greatly improves our chances of making a smooth transition.* By visiting, in imagination, the worlds which we may one day enter, we begin the process of transition in advance and reduce the chance that we shall be caught unawares.

At the same time, there is a limit to the amount of loss and change that we, or our patients, can take. We soon feel overwhelmed when we contemplate anything so enormous as the loss of a husband or wife or child, the effects of mutilating surgery, or the ending of our own lives. We need to find ways of distancing ourselves from the problems as well as ways of tackling them.

Confrontation and avoidance

It is easy for sociologists to write angrily about patients' "rights to know the truth" about their illnesses and to accuse doctors of obfuscation and deceit if they are not brutally frank. But doctors, who have the task of breaking bad news, know that this is never easy, for the doctor or the recipient. We try to find ways of mitigating the pain, and we rely on our own intuition to tell us whether or not we are telling too much or too little. People may have a "right to know" but there are times when they may also have a right not to know more than they can take.

One researcher who has studied this matter in some depth is Mardi Horowitz.[12] He points out that people faced with major psychological trauma need to find a balance between the intrusive images and thoughts which tend to force themselves painfully into consciousness and the avoidance of such thoughts by distraction or other psychological defences. He has developed a scale, the "impact of events scale", to measure these two tendencies.[13] Most people attempt to find a balance between confrontation and avoidance; they oscillate back and forth between the two and hope to find a way of gradually taking in and processing painful thoughts without becoming overwhelmed. But there is a minority who get stuck at one or other extreme of oscillation; Horowitz terms them "sensitisers" and "avoiders".

The allied concepts of "grief work" (Freud[14]) and "worry work" (Janis and Leventhal[15]) have been proposed to reflect the idea that *it takes time and effort to come to terms with painful realities* but that this is a job that is worth doing. The bereaved person cannot and does not have to grieve all the time nor does the dying patient have to spend all of his or her life preparing for death, but each needs to find a balance between confrontation and avoidance, grief and denial.

Preparing people for loss—breaking bad news

One way of coping is to divide the information that needs to be confronted into "bite sized chunks". Doctors do this when we break bad news a little at a time, telling a patient as much as we think he or she is able to take in. *Patients themselves seldom ask questions unless they are ready for the answers and will usually ask precisely what they want to know and no more*. It follows that we should invite questions and listen carefully to what is asked rather than assuming that we know what the patient is ready to know. By monitoring the input of information a person can control the speed with which they process that information and take the time that is needed if the internal changes are to keep pace with the external world.

The underlying problem can be summarised as follows: although a little anxiety puts us on our mettle and increases the rate and efficiency with which we process information, too much anxiety slows us down and impairs our ability to cope, our thought processes become disorganised, and we "go to pieces". It follows that *anything which enables us to keep anxiety within tolerable limits will help us to cope better with the process of change*. If we are breaking bad news it helps to do so in pleasant, home-like like surroundings and to invite the recipient to bring someone who can provide emotional support. A few minutes spent putting people at their ease and establishing a relationship of trust with them will not only make the whole experience less traumatic for them but it will increase their chance of taking in and making sense of the information which we then provide.

Confronting and avoiding loss

The essence of grief is the need to search for something or someone we have lost. This is seen most obviously in the young child separated from his or her mother who will cry aloud and search restlessly. In the statistically rare event that the person lost is dead or, for some other reason, unable to return, we are faced with the same need to search and to cry aloud but without hope that our cry will be answered.

As we shall see in the first chapter, which treats of bereavement by death, adults know such behaviour to be pointless but this does not prevent us from experiencing a powerful impulse to cry and to search. At the same time we experience a similarly powerful impulse to inhibit or avoid so irrational and antisocial a reaction.

Defence and coping

The outcome is a compromise. We adopt whatever means we have found most effective in the past and whatever techniques we have learned are proper to the occasion to cope with the situation. Psychiatrists describe a wide range of "defence mechanisms" having the effect of enabling us to distance ourselves from the painful realisation of loss. These include "denial" (denying the truth of a painful reality), "amnesia" (forgetting facts that we dare not remember), "dissociation" (numbing or other ways to shut out or confine mental pain), and the more obvious and conscious attempts to avoid or postpone talking or thinking about painful topics. Because most of these were first described in patients who were undergoing psychotherapy and because the repression and avoidance of traumatic memories has long been recognised as an occasional cause of psychiatric disorder there is a tendency to regard all such defensive behaviour as harmful.

In recent years, however, it has been recognised that intermittent avoidance of loss is a normal part of grieving. Problems tend to emerge if either the avoidance is too protracted and complete or the other extreme is reached when a person becomes totally obsessed and preoccupied with the expression of grief. Avoidance then is best seen as a means of coping which may or may not prove

9

helpful depending on the circumstances in which it takes place. *To cope effectively it seems important to find the right balance* between total absorption with grief to the exclusion of all other concerns and the indefinite postponement of the work of grieving.

In this book we shall find that different situations evoke different ways of coping. Social rituals such as funerals may provide social sanction for grief after a death, but there is no such ritual to help an amputee to cope with the grief he or she feels when losing a limb. Similarly, anger may be recognised as a reasonable and socially acceptable response to assault, murder, or manslaughter but it creates embarrassment if it interrupts a funeral and is deplored if it follows the birth of a baby. Many of the situations met with in medicine evoke grief without, at the same time, providing the rituals and other forms of support that would facilitate its expression. *Members of the medical profession may be the only people to hand who are in a position to understand and to give the support that is needed.*

The doctor as an agent of change

It follows from what has been said that medical practitioners are in a unique position to help people through the turning points in their lives which arise at times of loss. We are agents of change. To fulfil this role we need information and the skills to use it effectively.

One of our problems as care givers is our ignorance of our patients' views of the world. Not only do we seldom know what they know or think they know about the situation they face, we do not even know how that situation is going to change their lives. It follows that if we are to be of any help to them we should take the trouble to find out how they see the situation; we should then, when possible, add to their knowledge or correct any mis-perceptions, taking care to use language that they can understand. (This is easier said than done when words like "cancer" and "death" mean different things to doctors than they do to most patients.) Above all, we should be prepared to spend time helping them to talk through and to make sense of the implications of the information we have given. If possible, we should be prepared to see them several times to facilitate this process of growth and change. General practitioners, because they are likely to know the person well and to be in touch with them over time, are often well placed to provide this "trickle" of care.

When we do this we become facilitators of the process of transition. This is an important role to which insufficient attention has been paid in the past.

Outline of this book

It is the object of this book to point the way, and, like most signposts, we shall start at the end of the journey. We shall look first at the way in which people cope with two of the most common forms of major loss, the death of a spouse (chapter 2) and the loss of a child (chapter 3). The reason for placing bereavement near the start of the book is that it provides us with an unusually clear picture of the nature of grief and its consequences. We then go on to look at other life situations leading to separation from and the loss of loved people (chapter 4).

From loss of people we move on to look at the wider range of losses that arise when people who are moving from a state of health, in which they can take for granted the fact that their bodies and minds can be relied on to function in the accustomed ways, to states of non-health in which nothing can be taken for granted and they must lose parts of their bodies (chapter 5) or their sensory and cognitive functions (chapter 6). Though the grief which follows physical losses is different from the griefs which follow loss of a person, there are important similarities, and these situations teach us much about the process of adaptation which comes into play whenever one set of habitual assumptions must be abandoned and a new set learnt.

We broaden the frame of reference to include loss of occupations and other roles (chapter 7) followed by a scrutiny of some of the elusive forms of loss met with in medicine, which are often hidden or ignored (chapter 8).

Old age is a time when multiple losses of many types can occur. Brice Pitt's account expands many of the findings of earlier articles (chapter 9). This is followed by a consideration of the special problems that arise in the face of terminal illness in adults (chapter 10) and in children (chapter 11). We move on to consider the special problems posed by communal disasters (chapter 12) and the penultimate chapter (chapter 13) recognises that doctors themselves suffer grief and may need support if we are to continue to give support to others who are grieving. We hope that, by focusing on the griefs and psychosocial transitions that arise in each of these varied situations and circumstances, a coherent picture and plan will gradually emerge. The book is rounded off (chapter 14) with a review of the basic assumptions that can be made, in our present state of knowledge, about the psychology of loss and the principles of care that follow from these assumptions.

Recommended reading

Markus *et al* show how general practitioners can prevent mental illness and reduce psychological problems by recognising the losses that take place at each of the life stages and by giving appropriate support.[9] Marris adopts a sociological perspective to loss and change which shows how it influences the "structures of meaning" which govern our lives and social institutions.[16]

1 Clark S. *Loss and grief in general practice: a pilot study.* National Convention of the Royal Australian College of General Practitioners, 1986.
2 Parkes CM. *Bereavement: studies of grief in adult life.* 3rd ed. London: Tavistock/ Routledge, 1996 and Pelican: Harmondsworth, 1998.
3 Paykel ES. Life stress and psychiatric disorder. In: Dohrenwendt BS, Dohrenwendt BP, eds. *Stressful life events: their nature and effects.* New York: Wiley, 1974.
4 Clegg F. Grief and loss in elderly people in a psychiatric setting. In: Chigier E, ed. *Grief and mourning in contemporary society. Vol. 1. Psychodynamics.* London. Freund, 1988.
5 Burton R. *The anatomy of melancholy.* 11th ed. Amsterdam: Theatrum Orbis Terrarum, 1813.
6 Lindemann E. The symptomatology and management of acute grief. *Am J Psychiatry* 1944;**101**:141.
7 Aldrich CK. The dying patient's grief. *JAMA* 1963;**184**:329.
8 Ross EK. *On death and dying.* London: Tavistock, 1970.
9 Markus AC, Parkes CM, Tomson P, Johnstone M. *Psychological problems in general practice.* Oxford: Oxford University Press, 1989.
10 Parad HJ, Caplan G. A framework for studying families in crisis. In: Parad HJ, ed. *Crisis intervention: selected readings.* New York: Family Service Association of America, 1965.
11 Parkes CM. Psycho-social transitions: a field for study. *Soc Sci Med* 1971;**5**: 101–15.
12 Horowitz M. *Stress response syndromes.* Northvale, New Jersey: Aronson, Northvale, 1986.
13 Horowitz M, Wilner N, Alvarez W. Impact of event scale: measure of subjective stress. *Psychosom Med* 1979;**41**:209–18.

14 Freud S. Mourning and Melancholia. In: Strachey J, ed. *The standard edition of the complete psychological works of Sigmund Freud.* Vol 14. London: Hogarth Press, 1953.

15 Janis IL, Leventhal H. Psychological aspects of physical illness and hospital care. In: *Handbook of clinical psychology.* New York: McGraw Hill, 1965.

16 Marris P. *Loss and change.* London: Routledge and Kegan Paul, 1974.

2 Bereavement in adult life

COLIN MURRAY PARKES

The effects of bereavement on health

After a major loss, such as the death of a spouse or child, up to a third of those most directly affected will suffer detrimental effects on their physical or mental health, or both (see Jacobs for a recent review of the evidence[1]). Such bereavements increase the risk of death from heart disease and suicide as well as causing or contributing to a variety of psychosomatic and psychiatric disorders. About a quarter of widows and widowers will experience levels of depression and anxiety which meet strict criteria for psychiatric illness at some time during the first year of bereavement. The risk drops to about 17% by the end of the first year and continues to decline thereafter.

Assessing the risk

Much research in recent years has enabled us to identify people at special risk after bereavement either because the circumstances of the bereavement are unusually traumatic or because they are themselves already vulnerable. A knowledge of bereavement risk not only helps us to decide who needs care, it also helps us to decide what type of care is needed and to ensure that available resources are focused on the people who need them most. It follows that all who offer support to the bereaved should be aware of these factors and make use of them when deciding who should be advised

14

to seek counselling or other forms of help. Risk indicators are listed in box 2.1.

Box 2.1   Factors increasing the risk of bereavement

Traumatic circumstances

- Death of a spouse or child
- Death of a parent (particularly in early childhood or adolescence)
- Sudden, unexpected, and untimely deaths (particularly if associated with horrific circumstances)
- Multiple deaths (particularly disasters)
- Deaths by suicide
- Deaths by murder or manslaughter

Vulnerable people

General

- Low self esteem
- Low trust in others
- Previous psychiatric disorder
- Previous suicidal threats or attempts
- Absent or unhelpful family

Specific

- Ambivalent attachment to deceased person
- Dependent or interdependent attachment to deceased person
- Insecure attachment to parents in childhood (particularly learned fear and learned helplessness)

Traumatic bereavement

While most bereavements can be said to be traumatic some are more traumatic than others. It comes as no surprise to find that the deaths of partners and children carry more risk than the deaths of parents and siblings nor that unexpected and untimely deaths are more psychologically stressful than deaths that have been anticipated and prepared for. Multiple losses and deaths caused by human agency such as suicide and murder all increase the risk, although one should never assume that everyone who experiences such a loss will need help from outside the family. It follows that,

15

while the assessment of bereavement risk is important, we should consider the special circumstances of each case.

Vulnerability

to bereavement may be general or specific—that is, it may reflect a general vulnerability to all kinds of stress or a special sensitivity to bereavement.

General vulnerability

may be associated with a history of mental ill health, low self esteem, or lack of social support. Low self esteem reflects general feelings of insecurity.

Specific vulnerability

arises from the death of a person on whom the survivor has been dependent or with whom a highly ambivalent relationship existed. Previous unresolved grief from an earlier loss can sensitise people to the effects of later losses, and there are some dysfunctional families in which nobody can cope with loss.

Grief often reflects the nature of the attachment to the lost person, and this, in turn, may reflect earlier attachments in the person's life. These attachments reflect the parenting which the person received early in life and give rise to the basic assumptions which will colour that person's future relationships and self view. It is essential to our survival that we learn what to fear, and this simple fact makes it most important for children to be sensitive to the fears of their parents. If the parents are overanxious and see the world as a dangerous place and their children as extremely vulnerable we should not be surprised if the children grow up with a similar view of the world. Hence "learned fear" is a common cause of excessive fear and clinging after bereavements and other life stresses. Similarly, it is important for the developing child to learn how to cope, and there are some forms of parenting that undermine autonomy and give rise to "learned helplessness". These have been postulated as a common precursor of depressive reactions to stress and particularly to the loss of people on whom the bereaved have come to rely. (For a more detailed exposition of these views and of the evidence that underlies them see Parkes.[2])

Before we look more closely at some of the other problems of bereavement it will be useful to look at the normal course of grief.

This will provide us with a yardstick by which we can better understand the abnormal.

The components of grief

Three main components affect the process of grieving. Each of these is present throughout but is likely to be more obvious at different times in the course of grief. They include the conflicting urges to cry, to control crying, and to change.

The need to cry and search for the lost person

The most obvious and distinctive component is the urge to cry aloud and to search for the one who is lost. This "separation distress" reflects the emotional and behavioural reaction which takes places whenever we are separated, for any length of time, from those we love. It is part of the range of behavioural systems which, thanks to the work of John Bowlby and his colleagues, have become known as attachment behaviours and have given rise to attachment theory (Holmes gives a succinct review[3]).

According to this theory, in the environment in which humans evolved our survival depended on our ability to stay close to our living group and all separations were dangerous. In common with other social animals we evolved a repertoire of attachment behaviour which ensured that parents would stay close to children and eventually led to the complex network of attachments that comprise the family. Among the elements of attachment behaviour which have been studied are smiling, clinging, and following, all of which tend to maintain attachment, and crying and searching, which come into operation after separation. These behaviour patterns appear sequentially in the developing infant during the course of the first year of life and remain active throughout life.

Although rooted in instinct, they are modified by learning from their inception and remain open to modification. There is a tendency for patterns that have been established in childhood to influence the relationships which develop later in life but personal experience, family traditions, and the wider impact of culture and belief systems all influence attachment behaviour.

The need to inhibit and control crying

Almost the first thing a mother attempts to do is to persuade her baby not to cry, and this persuasion often goes beyond the succour that is the best and most satisfactory response to tears. Social influences continue to affect the expression of separation distress throughout life. This gives rise to a conflict between the deeply felt need to express grief and the powerful prohibitions which cause people to limit or inhibit this expression. The intelligent human adult knows that it is illogical, useless, and antisocial to wander the streets crying aloud for a dead person. Consequently bereaved people often try to avoid reminders of the loss and to suppress the expression of grief. What emerges is a compromise, a partial expression of feelings which are experienced as arising compellingly and illogically from within. Typically people oscillate back and forth between the "pangs of grief" in which they are preoccupied with thoughts of loss and give vent to tears and relatively calm periods during which they control tears and direct their thoughts to other matters. There is much empirical evidence that supports the claims of the psychoanalytic school that excessive repression of grief is harmful and can give rise to delayed and distorted grief. On the other hand, there is also evidence that people who go to the other extreme and become obsessively preoccupied with grieving are also likely to have persisting difficulties.[4]

Each culture has found its own "solution" to this conflict, some providing sanction for the expression of emotions and others expecting them to be strictly controlled. The decline in religious observance and belief in Western societies during the current century has been associated with increasing attenuation of mourning. There is some evidence from cross cultural studies that members of societies such as the Apache, who inhibit the expression of grief (N C Mintz, personal communication), may be more vulnerable to subsequent depression than societies such as those in the Caribbean, who encourage flamboyant grieving.[5]

The need to discover a new identity

It takes a long time for bereaved spouses to discover what changes in life are necessary and how their views of themselves and their world must change as they move from the world of the married to the world of the widow or widower. This process is similar to the relearning that takes place when a person suffers disablement or the loss of a body part, and we shall return to look more closely at the process in the chapter dealing with this problem (pp 47–56).

Suffice it to say that the loss of a loved person inevitably creates a host of discrepancies between our internal world and the world that now exists for us. This is not only true at the superficial level (Who will be there when I get in from work in the evening?) but also at the deeper level of basic assumptions (If I am no longer a married man, what am I?). Bereaved people are repeatedly surprised at the number of habits of thought which involve the other person and the extent to which things take their meaning from the presence of another person. Often the person who has died is the person we would have turned to at times of trouble and here we are, in the biggest trouble we have ever experienced, constantly turning towards someone who is not there. Small wonder that bereaved people often feel as if life itself has lost its meaning.

Both avoidance and preoccupation with loss make it difficult for people to accept the reality of what has happened. Until they have done that they are likely to find it difficult to review and revise their basic assumptions about themselves and the place in the world which now exists for them.

The course of grief

These components of grief interact to produce a changing pattern. Although the moment of death is usually a time of great distress, this is usually quickly repressed and, in Western society, the impact is soon followed by a period of numbness which lasts for hours or days. This is sometimes referred to as *the first phase of grieving*.[6] It is soon followed by the *second phase*, intense feelings of pining for the lost person accompanied by intense anxiety. These "pangs of grief" are transient episodes of separation distress between which the bereaved person continues to engage in the normal functions of eating, sleeping, and carrying out essential responsibilities in an apathetic and anxious way.

All appetites are diminished, weight is lost, concentration and short term memory are diminished, and as time goes by the bereaved person often becomes irritable and depressed, giving rise to the *third phase* of grieving, disorganisation, and despair. Many find themselves going over the events which led up to the loss

19

again and again as if, even now, they could find out what went wrong and put it right. The memory of the dead person is never far away and about half of widows report *hypnagogic hallucinations* in which, at times of drowsiness or relaxation, they see or hear the dead person near at hand. These hallucinations are distinguished from the hallucinations of psychosis by the circumstances in which they arise and by their transience—they disappear as soon as the bereaved arouse themselves. A sense of the dead person near at hand is also common and may persist.

As time passes the intensity and frequency of the pangs of grief tend to diminish, although they often return with renewed intensity at anniversaries and other occasions which bring the dead person strongly to mind. Consequently *the phases of grief should not be regarded as a rigid sequence that is passed through only once*. The bereaved person must pass back and forth between pining and despair many times before they come to the *final phase* of reorganisation, and even then people will often find themselves experiencing another pang.

After a major loss such as the death of a loved spouse or partner most people will recognise that they are recovering at some time in the course of the second year. The appetite for food is often the first appetite to return, perhaps because starvation promotes appetite. By the third or fourth month of bereavement the weight that was lost initially has usually returned and by the sixth month many people have put on too much weight. It may be many more months before people begin to care about their appearance, sexual and social appetites return, and they feel motivated to lose weight again.

Complicated grief

Bereavement, as we have seen, has profound effects on the emotions, and these are accompanied by equally profound physiological effects. Research has shown that the immune response system is temporarily impaired,[7,8] and endocrine changes such as increased adrenocortical activity and increases in serum concentrations of prolactin and growth hormone occur as in other situations which evoke depression and distress.[1] These may account for some of the effects of bereavement on physical health.

Various psychiatric disorders can also be caused by bereavement, the commonest being clinical depression, anxiety states, panic

---

Box 2.2   Complications of bereavement

Physical

- Impairment of immune response system
- Increased adrenocortical activity
- Increased serum prolactin
- Increased growth hormone
- Psychosomatic disorders
- Increased mortality from heart disease (especially in elderly widowers)

Psychiatric

Non-specific

- Depression (with or without suicide risk)
- Anxiety/panic disorders
- Other psychiatric disorders

Specific

- Post-traumatic stress disorder
- Delayed or inhibited grief
- Chronic grief

---

syndromes, and post-traumatic stress disorder. These often coexist and overlap with each other as they do with the more specific morbid grief reactions. These last disorders are of special interest because they help to explain why some people come through bereavement unscathed or strengthened and matured by the experience while others "break down".

It is a paradox that some people who cope with bereavement by repressing the expression of grief are more likely to break down later than are people who burst into tears. They are more liable to suffer sleep disorders, episodes of depression, and hypochondriacal symptoms resembling the symptoms of the illness that caused the bereavement ("identification symptoms"). Not all psychogenic symptoms, however, are a consequence of repressed or avoided grief; some reflect the loss of security which often follows a major loss and causes people to misinterpret as sinister the normal symptoms of anxiety and tension.

At the other end of the spectrum of morbid grief are people who express intense distress before and after bereavement. Subsequently they cannot stop grieving and go on to suffer from Chronic Grief. This may reflect a dependent or pseudoindependent relationship with the dead person or it may follow the loss of someone who was ambivalently loved. In the former case, the bereaved person cannot believe that he or she can survive without the support of the person on whom they had depended. In the latter, their grief is complicated by mixed feelings of anger and guilt which make it difficult for them to stop punishing themselves ("Why should I be happy now that my partner is dead?").

These two patterns of grieving often seem to occur in the "avoiders" and "sensitisers" described on pp 7–8.

Prevention and treatment of complicated grief

It follows that much can be done to reduce the risk of complicated bereavement by providing support to patients and their families before a death occurs, and this will be considered in detail in chapters 10 and 11.

Some degree of ambivalence is present in all relationships. Its effects can be assuaged if the person has had the opportunity to say, "I'm sorry", and to make restitution by giving conscientious and devoted care during the course of the last illness. Many people will say of such times, "We were never closer." If the family have been encouraged and supported so that they have been able to carry out their duty of care and the death has been peaceful, anger and guilt are much less likely to complicate the course of grieving.

Members of health care teams are often in a position to prepare people for the losses that are to come by including them when bad news is broken and supporting them in much the same way that we support the patient (see pp 8–9). We are also likely to be present when, or soon after, people die and can do a great deal to support bereaved families at this time. We shall be more likely to succeed in this if we have already established a relationship of trust with the person. Newly bereaved people often feel and behave, for a while, like frightened and helpless children and will respond best to the kind of support that is normally given by a parent. This is not the time to hold back, and a touch or a hug will often do more to facilitate grieving than any words that we can utter.

How does this affect staff?

A visit from the general practitioner to the family home on the day after a death has occurred will enable us to reinforce this support and to answer any questions about the death and its causes that may still be troubling the family. This is a time of great bewilderment, and simple instructions about the death certification process together with reassurance that nothing has to be done in a hurry will help.

Those who have experienced a great loss lose any sense of security they may have had in the past. The world has become a dangerous place in which there is disaster round every corner. Consequently they may feel under great pressure to take action to ward off further dangers. Gentle reassurance that there is very little that they need to do at this time and that it is better not to make important decisions which they might later regret is often wise. When possible people may need to be relieved of major responsibilities so that they have time and space for grieving. Maybe family members and friends can share in the care of the children and employers permit a period of compassionate leave.

This does not mean that bereaved people should be relieved of all responsibilities. They will need things to do and can be encouraged to take part in planning the funeral and consulted on all matters relevant to the death. This is a time when the dead often receive more attention than the living and we need to recognise that fact.

During the next few weeks bereaved people need the support of those they can trust. We can often reassure them of the normality of grief, explain the symptoms to which it gives rise, and show by our own behaviour and attitudes that it is permissible to express grief. If we feel moved to tears at such times there is no harm in showing it. Bereaved people may need reassurance that they are not going mad if they "break down", that the frightening symptoms of anxiety and tension are not signs of mortal illness, and that they are not letting the side down if they withdraw, for a while, from their accustomed tasks.

As time passes people may also need permission to take a break from grieving. They cannot grieve all the time and may need permission to return to work or do other things that enable them to escape, for a while, from grief. It is only if they get the balance wrong that difficulties are likely to ensue.

The first anniversary is often a time of renewed grieving, but thereafter the need to stop grieving and move forward in life may

23

create a new set of problems. People may need reassurance that their duty to the dead is done and encouragement to face the world that is now open to them. For the faint hearted this can be hard, and they may be tempted to cling to their grief as an excuse to remain shut off from life. For them, *the most important thing we have to offer is our confidence in their personal worth and strength.* We should beware of becoming the "strong" doctor who will look after the "weak" patient for ever, but this does not mean that we should become angry and dismissive, reprimanding the patient for becoming "dependent". We must understand the bereaved person's fears without sharing them; it is our faith in their strength not our contempt for their weakness that will get them through.

For bereaved people who have lost confidence in themselves it takes real courage to go to a supermarket, invite someone to dinner, or do many of the things that, in the long run, will get them out of the rut of depression and withdrawal. We can help them to set targets for themselves and, when they achieve these targets, we can applaud their efforts. They deserve it, and we are likely to be the only people, apart from the bereaved themselves, who understand how hard it has been. Once people begin to make progress it is often they who will suggest the next target. *Nothing succeeds like success*, and it is good to see the "little woman" or the "helpless man" beginning to discover the real talents and strengths that they possess.

In the end most bereaved people come through the experience stronger and wiser than they went into it. It is rewarding to see them through.

If the process gets stuck we need to consider why.

Is this person suffering from clinical depression or post-traumatic stress disorder (PTSD)?

In either case an antidepressant such as fluoxetine may be needed (but note that bereaved people who are depressed may be at risk of suicide, and it may be dangerous to prescribe the more cardiotoxic antidepressants). The management of post-traumatic stress disorder will be discussed in more detail on pp 118–9 and 123–4.

Have we failed to recognise that some earlier grief has been aroused by this one?

May be a course of psychotherapy would help the person to deal with this earlier loss, and there are some professional counsellors with the necessary skills (although buried griefs of this kind are likely to fall outside the expertise of the average volunteer counsellor or mutual help group).

Is there a self punitive element in the grieving?

Confession may or may not be good for the soul but it is certainly good for the psyche, and bereaved people often benefit from sharing feelings of guilt and examining their implications with an accepting and non-judgmental counsellor. It is of little use to contradict these utterances (one should never tell people that they should not feel emotions, however illogical these may seem), rather we can help by challenging them to find a constructive use for feelings that easily become destructive ("If that's how you feel, what are you going to do about it" is often a better response than, "You shouldn't blame yourself").

Are the bereaved caught in a vicious circle?

Fear or anxiety may have produced bodily symptoms that have evoked more fear thereby aggravating the situation or family members may be frightening each other and creating alarm which feeds into a belief that another disaster is looming. Anything which breaks the vicious circle, from emotional support and reassurance to breathing or relaxation exercises or a short course of an anxiolytic drug, will switch the bereaved into a de-escalating cycle which brings the problem to an end. But note, one study of patients referred to a programme for withdrawal of benzodiazepines showed that no less than 20% had started taking the drug after a bereavement.[9]

Have we failed to recognise a physical illness requiring treatment?

There is little doubt that bereavement can aggravate a number of physical complaints, particularly in older people, and it is unwise to assume that all of the symptoms which follow bereavement are psychological in origin. Even if the result is negative a careful physical examination will usually reassure us and the patient that all is well. We need to look out for signs of heart disease, and there is evidence of increased mortality from myocardial infarction and arteriosclerotic heart disease during the first 3 months after the death of a wife and, to a lesser extent, husband. In the event that there is a history or ongoing evidence of coronary impairment a β blocker may be considered as a means of reducing the damaging influence of emotions on the heart. Older people often suffer aggravation of symptoms of muscle and joint conditions.

Summary

Bereavement teaches us that when faced with a loss most people need permission and encouragement to grieve, but they may also need permission and encouragement in due time to stop grieving and get on with their lives. It takes sensitivity and tact to know which.

For most bereaved people the natural and most effective form of help will come from their own families, and only about a third of those who suffer a major loss will need extra help from outside. But the modern nuclear family is often dispersed; its members may prove unhelpful and may even block a person's attempts to grieve. At such times help from outside the family may make a crucial difference, and *random allocation studies of widows at risk indicate that the right help given to the right people at the right time can reduce that risk* (for further details see Parkes[2]).

In Western countries men often need help in expressing grief whereas women, who are more in touch with their emotions than men, may need help with reviewing and replanning their lives. Men are more vulnerable to inhibited or avoided grief and have a higher mortality from heart disease. Women, on the other hand, are more likely to seek psychiatric help for affective disorders and chronic grief than men (Stroebe and Stroebe review this evidence[4]).

In the acute stages it is usually best to provide individual support by personal contact, preferably in the person's home. Later, the help of a group in which bereaved participants can learn from each other as well as from a counsellor is likely to be appropriate. Organisations such as Cruse Bereavement Care and the member organisations of the National Association of Bereavement Services may be able to provide either of these types of help. The Compassionate Friends (for bereaved parents), Lesbian and Gay Bereavement, Support after Murder and Manslaughter (SAMM), and the Widow-to-Widow programmes, which exist in the United States and other parts of the world, provide mutual help by bereaved people for others with the same types of bereavement. Further details of these and other organisations are given in the appendix.

Members of the caring professions are often in a position to offer help to the bereaved and have a great deal to offer but bereavements are so common and the need so great that we should beware of offering more help than we can deliver. If we can work as members of a team, drawing support from each other and making use, when appropriate, of the other sources of help that exist outside the health care team, we shall be much less likely to find ourselves overburdened with the griefs of our patients and their families and will continue to find this work rewarding.

Recommended reading

Jacobs gives a good account of the physiological and psychological effects of bereavement on health.[1] Parkes expands the argument of this chapter and provides its scientific basis,[2] and Parkes, Relf, and Couldrick provide an outline of the principles and practice of counselling in terminal care and bereavement.[10]

1 Jacobs S. *Pathologic grief: maladaptation to loss.* Washington, DC: American Psychiatric Press, 1993.
2 Parkes CM. *Bereavement: studies of grief in adult life.* 3rd ed. London: Tavistock/ Routledge, 1996 and Pelican: Harmondsworth, 1998.
3 Holmes J. *John Bowlby & attachment theory.* London: Routledge, 1993.
4 Stroebe W, Stroebe MS. *Bereavement and health: the psychological and physical consequences of partner loss.* Cambridge: Cambridge University Press, 1987.
5 Burgoine E. A cross-cultural comparison of bereavement among widows in New Providence, Bahamas, and London, England. London: International Conference on Grief and Bereavement in Contemporary Society, July 1988.
6 Bowlby J, Parkes CM. Separation and loss within the family. In: Anthony EJ, ed. *The child in his family.* New York: Wiley, 1970.
7 Bartrop RW, Lazarus L, Luckhurse E, *et al.* Depressed lymphocyte function after bereavement. *Lancet.* 1977;**i**:834–6.
8 Schleiffer SJ, Keller SE, Camerino M, *et al.* Suppression of lymphocyte stimulation following bereavement, *JAMA.* 1983;**250**:374–7.
9 Hamlin M, Hammersley D. Benzodiazepines following bereavement. London: International Conference on Grief and Bereavement in Contemporary Society, July 1988.
10 Parkes CM, Relf M, Couldrick A. Counselling in terminal care and bereavement. In: Davis H, ed. *Communication and counselling in health care.* Leicester: BPS Books, 1996.

3 Bereavement in childhood

DORA BLACK

The effects of loss on children depend on their age and developmental level, their prior relationship with the lost one, whether they were prepared for the loss, and their subsequent experiences, including the reaction of those around them and the opportunity to receive counselling.

In this chapter we examine the way in which attachments develop and the consequences when they come to an end. We focus on bereavement by death. Other types of loss in childhood will be considered in later chapters.

The development of attachment bonds

Infants do not come into the world as "empty slates" but bring with them complex behavioural systems which have evolved through natural selection. One system which has been well studied protects the child from danger during the long period of extrauterine immaturity. It involves the development of mutual attachment behaviour which ensures that the child does not stray far from a care taker. The infant is an active partner in the development of this behaviour, using instinctive behaviours to engage a care taker in protection. These include smiling, vocalising, crying, and, later, returning frequently to the secure base of the adult after exploratory forays.[1] Infant attachment is at its height at about 3 years of age and then becomes increasingly diffused by the development of other relationships, but it remains an important behavioural system throughout life, later relationships qualitatively echoing the earlier ones.

Box 3.1 Components of attachment behaviour in infants

Behaviour maintaining attachment

- Smiling
- Vocalising (babbling)
- Clinging
- Following

Behaviour on separation

- Crying (protest)
- Restless searching
- High anxiety
- Irritability

For optimal emotional, social, and psychosexual development to occur, children need a warm, secure, affectionate, individualised, and continuous experience of care from a few care takers who interact with them in a sensitive way and who can live in harmony with each other.

Parents, especially the mother, make space in their minds for their child even before birth, developing what Winnicott called "primary maternal preoccupation"[2] in later pregnancy and bringing to the early relationship with their infant their own experiences of being parented (of secure or insecure attachment) which influence the pattern of care they give in their turn. The relationships which are created are dynamic ones, each influencing the other and in turn being influenced by other past and current relationships.[3]

Separation and loss in childhood

Infants and toddlers react to separation from an attachment figure by protesting vigorously. If their cries are not successful in restoring the adult, protest eventually gives way to despair, and, eventually, if they are not restored to their attachment figure, pathological states of detachment and indifference may ensue. They probably have little concept of death, and their reactions to the disappearance of a parent from whatever cause are similar. Thus, a parent away for a few hours and one absent for longer evoke the same separation anxiety in infants and toddlers older than a few weeks or months.[4] Even very young children can mourn for a lost parent, although the form of their grief differs from that of adults and older children.[4,5] Their reactions tend to be bodily ones such as feeding difficulties, bed wetting, constipation, and sleeping difficulties.

By 5 years of age, most children can understand the difference between a separation (such as that caused by mother going into hospital or to visit a sick relative) which is temporary and death, which means permanent separation. They know that death is irreversible, universal, has a cause, involves permanent separation, and that dead people differ from live people in a number of respects. They are immobile, unfeeling, cannot hear, see, smell, or speak. All their bodily functions cease, and they do not require sustenance. It is more difficult for them to understand that dead people change in their appearance, and this concept does not develop until nearer puberty.[6]

Children from 5–11 years are more likely to be able to comprehend the physical changes death brings and are helped by being able to perceive these changes for themselves. They should be told what to expect and then, if they agree, be allowed to view the body. Exceptions to this rule may arise if the body is severely mutilated or the child or parents have a strong aversion to the idea of viewing. In such cases additional support may be needed.

Their characteristic response to the death of a parent is an increase in activity, and behavioural problems may result. Hallucinations of the dead person are a common feature of grief in adult life (see p 20). They can also be experienced by young children who may interpret them as evidence of parental return or as evidence of persecution by the ghost of the dead parent because of imagined shortcomings on the part of the child, giving rise to severe anxiety. Because of their need for parenting, children who lose one parent often become very anxious about the survival of the other and may protect that parent from knowledge of their own distress. That, and the difficulty of sustaining sad affects, may lead the parent or teacher to believe that the child has recovered from or has not been affected by a bereavement.

Reactions to bereavement in childhood

The florid reactions tend not to last beyond a few weeks, with most children regaining their previous level of psychosocial functioning.[7] As assessed by parental reports, however, children have higher levels of emotional disturbance and symptoms than non-bereaved children for up to 2 years and up to 40% of bereaved children are symptomatic at 1 year.[8,9] In their direct assessments of bereaved children Weller and colleagues found that 37% of their sample of 38 bereaved prepubertal children suffered from a major depressive disorder a year after bereavement.[10]

Longing for reunion is common and may lead to suicidal thoughts in bereaved children and adolescents, although they are rarely acted on.[10] Other difficulties include problems with learning and failure to maintain progress at school.[11]

Long term effects of bereavement on children

Children who are bereaved early are more likely to develop psychiatric disorders in later childhood.[12] Rutter found that there was a fivefold increase in childhood psychiatric disorder in bereaved children compared with the general population.[13]

Adults who lost a parent in childhood seem to be more vulnerable than the general population to psychiatric disorder,[14,15] particularly depression and anxiety, and this is often precipitated by further losses. Attempted suicide is more common in adults bereaved in childhood.[16]

Children who lose their mother suffer a reduction in the quantity as well as quality of care, and this may account for the finding that they are differentially affected according to the sex of the deceased parent.[10]

Effects of the death of a sibling

There are fewer studies of loss of a sibling than of a parent. One study of 28 children found that 2 or 3 years after the death a high proportion of the children were emotionally or behaviourally disturbed and had a low self esteem.[17] If the child had been prepared for the sibling's death, had participated in the patient's care, and had been able to take leave of him or her and joined in the community rituals the outcome seemed to be better. The cost

31

to the survivor of having to carry all the parental expectations may be great.

As with the death of a parent, the reactions to a sibling's death depend on the developmental stage of the child and the prior relationship. Children compete for parental attention and often feel resentful of the attention given to a sick sibling, especially if they feel deprived because of the needs of that child, which may include a parent in attendance at hospital. Guilt may be the predominant emotion which follows triumph at having survived when a sibling dies. Young children may believe that their hostile or ambivalent feelings actually caused their sibling's death, and this may lead to profound behavioural changes. If the sibling was an older one and carried out some parental functions the reaction may be similar to that described after parental loss.

Helping bereaved children

Children are rarely prepared for the death of a parent or a sibling and yet we know from studies of bereaved adults that mourning is aided by a foreknowledge of the imminence and inevitability of death.[18] If children are forewarned they have lower levels of anxiety than those who are not, even within the same family.[19] Practitioners attending a dying parent can help the other parent to understand the necessity of preparing the children and help them to pick the right time to do so. Even so, it is difficult for young children to summon up images of the lost parent or to anticipate situations which might remind them of him or her. While an adult or adolescent could prepare for pain on revisiting the site of a previously shared activity, such preparation is not available to a child without adult intervention.

Others have set up programmes offering group meetings for bereaved children on the premise that it is helpful for children to know that others are similarly affected by bereavement,[20] but this intervention has not been evaluated.

The general practitioner or other member of the primary care team can monitor the bereaved child to ensure the care he or she is receiving is optimal. This may involve arranging periods of relief from the company of a grief stricken bereaved or widowed parent, advice about how to cope with other children's questions and adults' expressions of condolence, factual information about the cause of death and the processes of death, burial, and cremation,

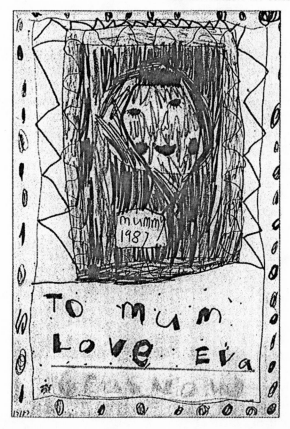

Figure 3.1 Asked to draw her mother as she imagined she might be after radiotherapy for carcinoma of the breast, 6 year old Eva at first drew mother with a scarf to hide her bald head and then attempted to hide the scarf in a similar coloured background. Subsequently she filled in the background with black and drew the "tombstone" below. Although she had not been told directly that mother was dying, she showed her therapist that she was aware of the likely future for her mother.

and advice to the carers about viewing the body,[21] attending the funeral,[22] returning to school, and promoting healthy mourning.

Young children in particular need the concrete experience of seeing the parent after death and having demonstrated to them the reality of death. Bereaved adults find it particularly difficult to help a child in this way, and the general practitioner could offer to accompany the child to the chapel of rest. Similarly, children benefit from attending the funeral but need some protection from the raw expressed grief common at that time. Attendance in the

33

company of someone less affected by the death than the immediate relatives is desirable. This could be the child's teacher or someone from the family practice with whom he or she is familiar.

The monitoring of and help with practical matters (applying for a home help, mobilising family support, ensuring adequate income, etc.) need to be accompanied by specific bereavement counselling for both child and surviving parent. A controlled trial of family therapy with children bereaved of a parent showed that the morbidity after bereavement of 40% at 1 year could be reduced to 20% by six sessions of family meetings which focused on promoting shared grief and mourning within the family and encouraging communication about the dead parent.[8,9] This study is currently being replicated to compare family and parental counselling.

Furman, a psychoanalyst, has described her sensitive work with individual children, which while not controlled gives pointers to the problems bereavement poses for children and how they can be helped.[5] The provision of preventive counselling intervention is properly the responsibility of the primary care team, by using, as necessary, the resources of national voluntary organisations (see appendix) such as Cruse Bereavement Care or local bereavement counselling services.

Finally, the practitioner needs to be aware of the small number of children who may need more specialised help in recovering from depressive or other symptoms which may be associated with bereavement. These will include children who may have been partly instrumental in causing death (of a sibling perhaps), sudden and particularly traumatic bereavements, children who have suffered more than one bereavement, adolescents who express suicidal ideas, and children who do not respond to the initial preventive interventions.

Recommended reading

Cruse Bereavement Care (see appendix) publishes useful literature for bereaved children and their carers and provides training and bereavement counselling services. Dyregrov's excellent handbook[23] for adults deserves a place in a practice library, and work books for primary school children can aid those counselling them.[24,25]

1 Bowlby J. *A secure base*. London: Routledge, Kegan Paul, 1988.
2 Winnicott D. *Through paediatrics to psychoanalysis*. London: Tavistock, 1958.
3 Reder P, Lucey C, eds. *Assessment of parenting*. London: Routledge, 1995.
4 Bowlby J. *Attachment and loss*. Vols 1–3. London: Hogarth Press, 1969–80.
5 Furman E. *A child's parent dies*. New Haven: Yale University Press, 1974.
6 Lansdown R, Benjamin G. The development of the concept of death in children aged 5–9 years. *Child Care Health Dev* 1985;**11**:13–20.
7 Fristad MA, Jedel R, Weller RA, *et al* Psychosocial functioning in children after the death of a parent. *Am J Psychiatry* 1993;**150**:511–3.
8 Black D, Urbanowicz MA. Bereaved children-family intervention. In: Stevenson JE, ed. *Recent research in developmental psychopathology*. Oxford: Pergammon, 1985:179–87.
9 Black D, Urbanowicz MA. Family intervention with bereaved children. *J Child Psychol Psychiatry* 1987;**28**:467–76.
10 Weller RA, Weller EB, Fristad MA, *et al*. Depression in recently bereaved prepubertal children. *Am J Psychiatry* 1991;**148**:1536–40.
11 Van Eerdewegh MM, Bieri MD, Parrilla RH, *et al* The bereaved child. *Br J Psychiatry* 1982;**140**:23–9.
12 Black D. Annotation: the bereaved child. *J Child Psychol Psychiatry* 1978;**19**:287–92.
13 Rutter M. *Children of sick parents*. Oxford: Oxford University Press, 1966.
14 Birtchnell J. Early parent death and mental illness. *Br J Psychiatry* 1970;**116**:281–8.
15 Brown GW, Harris T, Copeland JR. Depression and loss. *Br J Psychiatry* 1971;**130**:1–18.
16 Birtchnell J. The relationship between attempted suicide, depression and parent death. *Br J Psychiatry* 1970;**116**:307–13.
17 Pettle Michael SA, Lansdown RG. Adjustment to the death of a sibling. *Arch Dis Child* 1986;**61**:278–83.
18 Parkes CM. *Bereavement: studies of grief in adult life*. Harmondsworth: Penguin, 1986.
19 Rosenheim E, Reicher R. Informing children about a parent's terminal illness. *J Child Psychol Psychiatry* 1985;**26**:995–8.
20 Fleming S, Balmer L. Group intervention with bereaved children. In: Papadatou D, Papadatos C, eds. *Children and death*. Washington: Hemisphere, 1991.
21 Cathcart F. Seeing the body after death [editorial]. *BMJ* 1988;**297**:997–8.
22 Weller EB, Weller RA, Fristad MA, *et al*. Should children attend their parent's funeral? *J Am Acad Child Adolesc Psychiatry* 1988;**27**:559–62.
23 Dyregrov A. *Grief in childhood; a handbook for adults*. London: Jessica Kingsley, 1991.
24 Heegaard M. *When someone very special dies—children can learn to cope with grief*. Minneapolis, Woodland Press, 1991.
25 Heegaard M. *When something terrible happens: children can learn to cope with grief*. Minneapolis, Woodland Press, 1991.

4 Separation and related problems of pair bond relationships

ROBERT S. WEISS

Relationships of attachment

Marriages and similar relationships—all the strong pair bonds between adults, regardless of marital status—are not only partnerships in the management of personal and familial life but also adult attachments. They provide each of the partners with an emotional base with which is associated a sense of security and place.

Relationships of attachment arise as a result of complex interactions between each participant's perceptions of the other and each participant's earlier experiences in attachments to parents. These earlier experiences of attachments, together with hopes and fears to which they have contributed, arise anew in the early stages of an adult pair bond. They are then modified, for good or ill, as the relationship progresses. In the relationship's early days, the partners were likely to have been buoyed by a sense of comfort and completion when with the other. Each will have learned to associate the other's image and voice with feelings of security and wellbeing. If the marriage is reasonably happy, simply hearing the other's voice in a telephone call, or seeing the other's image in a photograph, will foster feelings of wellbeing. Furthermore, each will have become highly attuned to the other's rhythms of thought and feeling and each will have learned to be quickly responsive to the other's emotional tone. As a result interaction with the other can sustain each partner's steady functioning.

Problems in relationships

Problems can arise for various reasons. Sometimes the attachment of one or both partners is a reflection of an earlier attachment that was insecure and fostered distrust. When problems arise, as they will in all our lives, the partners may make negative assumptions about each other that belong properly to these earlier relationships rather than to the present situation. Alternatively a new partner may be blamed for failing to live up to idealised expectations, perhaps that the partner will remedy earlier losses and disappointments.

Whatever the cause, *marital problems are devastating in their effects because the relationship that should foster security instead becomes a source of threat.* The home base that should constitute a refuge becomes dangerous, a place in which it is necessary to be on guard. Conversation is defensive, each partner protecting the self against an expected assault. Interaction, instead of stabilising functioning, burdens it. Each partner is angry at the other for actual and potential attack. Each partner is also angry because the other is seen to be refusing the reassurance he or she might give just by being attentive and caring.

Such anger can express itself in nagging and sniping or in angry words and shouts. It can lead to thrown objects and blows. But almost always, even when anger explodes into blind rage, there are other elements also being expressed by words and actions, including the despair of isolation, a fear of the other's ability to hurt, and a misguided belief that the other can be intimidated or argued or shamed into becoming the loving figure of the relationship's earlier days.

Unhappiness in marriage need not have overt expression. In many unhappy relationships conflict is limited and instead one or both partners withhold love. Should the couple find themselves in the same room, each may inflict "the silent treatment" on the other. At the same time, each is likely to be made tense by awareness of the other's unexpressed anger. In such marriages each partner can feel utterly alone in the world: isolated within the marriage, prevented by the marriage from forming a new relationship of attachment, and unwilling to burden friends or family with admissions of unhappiness.

Symptomatic expressions of a marriage in which mutual anger has become embedded include tension, preoccupation, and bitter

37

hopelessness. If the couple are seen together by a doctor in connection with a child's illness, one may talk with, perhaps, an undertone of complaint; the other may sit silently, as though unconnected with what is being said. A truly unhappy couple may not divulge just how bad things are without sensitive, sympathetic interviewing; each partner feels there is too much chance of being misunderstood. Yet it will be found that the couple no longer kiss, perhaps no longer eat together. It will be difficult for such a couple to help each other to treat an ill child; the spirit of cooperation necessary for working together is absent.

Children and marital conflict

The child of an unhappy marriage is likely to be aware of the parents' distance from each other and their underlying anger. Some unhappily married parents do seem able, at least to an extent, to conceal from a child their feelings about each other and to show interest in and affection for the child. Usually, however, such parents have too little energy and too much preoccupation with the unhappy marriage and its effects on themselves to attend reliably and sensitively to the child's needs for secure attachment.

In general, *children do not do well when their parents are unhappy with each other.* There can be exceptional situations, including those in which the parents are successful in keeping their unhappiness to themselves and also those in which each parent respects the other's positive relationship with the child. But more common are situations in which one or both of the parents establishes an alliance with a child from which the other parent is excluded. While a development of this sort can sometimes foster early maturation in the child, it always involves emotional cost to the child. Most often it imposes on the child impossible dilemmas of maintaining incompatible loyalties and unrealisable commitments.

With or without such developments children whose parents are preoccupied by their unhappy marriage are likely to feel isolated. They can express this through withdrawal, in aberrant behaviour, or in commitment to a sustaining peer group. Once in a while a child with talent will escape a troubled home through success in school that brings with it recognition and approval or a child who is resilient or simply fortunate will find adult support outside the family. Most children in unhappy homes must make do as best they can with too little emotional and moral sustenance.

38

Helping troubled marriages

A couple whose relationship is troubled probably cannot be helped in a single session in their doctor's office. Rather, they are likely to need marital counselling that will extend over a number of sessions. If such counselling is available, the doctor might tactfully explore with the couple their willingness to work toward improving their marital partnership. Both partners are likely to recognise that they would be happier if their relationship were more satisfactory. And, if there are children, the children's wellbeing provides a powerful incentive for improving the relationship. Often, however, both partners have learned to live with things as they are and to believe that trying for change will only make matters worse. If marital counselling seems appropriate the doctor may have to be strongly supportive of it to overcome the couple's reluctance to accept the risks that counselling may seem to hold.

Yet the doctor should be careful not to insist too strongly that the couple seek counselling lest such insistence alienate them and also provide them with new reasons for mutual disappointment.

Marital separation

Should the couple give up on their relationship, both partners are likely to experience some form of separation distress. Each can, indeed, experience severe grief because of loss of the marriage, with all grief's symptoms of obsessive review and difficulties in sleeping. But, *unlike the grief which follows a loss by death, the grief of marital break up is likely to be confused, mixed with intense anger, and associated with uncertainties about personal acceptability and worth.*

Pair bond attachment, as was noted earlier, involves the incorporation of the other within the emotional system that fosters feelings of security. Ending a relationship of attachment, even one that was deeply troubled, triggers emergency reactions, including compulsion to regain the other, that occur whenever the attachment system is threatened. For a time the partners may each experience an anxious, driving preoccupation with regaining the other, a preoccupation that can coexist with intense anger and determination to be rid of the other. This ambivalence can be expressed in, for example, a telephone call that is reassuring because of the connection to the other but which then becomes a vehicle for berating the other. Ambivalence can also give rise to severe mood swings from elation at having achieved freedom to despair at the hopelessness of the situation. These mood swings add to the separated person's confusion and self doubt.

Ending a marriage also brings loss of familiar routines and change in social role to that of unattached person. Friends may take sides or may back off from both sides, leaving one or both partners socially adrift. Some degree of social isolation may persist for a year or more after separation.

Ending other serious relationships

All the consequences of the ending of a marriage or marriage-like relationship, with the possible exception of changes in social role, are also experienced by those who were in other relationships of attachment. While we have no single term in ordinary use to characterise non-marital relationships of attachment, we do have many ways of communicating whether a relationship is one of attachment or not. For example, a young woman might deny that a relationship is one of attachment by saying, "He's just a friend", or acknowledge that it is by saying, "We're partners". We have these linguistic devices for indicating that a relationship is or is not an attachment because the issue is of such emotional importance. An unmarried attached couple who end their relationship, whether they had been living together or not, are likely to experience the same distress, in all its bewildering manifestations, as a separating married couple.

Whether marital or not, the ending of pair bonds gives rise to anxiety, desire to re-establish the relationship coexisting with distrust of the relationship, and persisting tension likely to express itself in preoccupation and in sleep difficulties. Nor is the ending of a non-marital union necessarily easier than ending a marriage. While the ending of a marriage brings about a changed social status, the ending of a non-marital union may or may not do so. Endings that are little noted by others may foster feelings that others are uncaring and that the distress of the ending has to be dealt with alone.

Children and separation

Parents experiencing the separation distress that accompanies the voluntary ending of any pair bond are likely to have little energy for attending to the needs of their children. *The children of a couple who are breaking up, however, will inescapably be distressed and in need of parental attention.* They are likely to grieve the departure from their homes of one of their parents, to worry about the wellbeing of both parents, and to worry about their own wellbeing. If they are 9 or 10 or older they may express anger with one or both of their parents, despite their continued need for both parents' caring support. Their schoolwork is likely to suffer as they become preoccupied with their familial situation. Most at risk of negative consequences are those children who are "put in the middle" through being recruited as allies by one or both parents, used by one or both parents as messengers to the other parent, or asked by one or both parents to report on the other parent's activities.

Helping at the time of breakup

People going through separation must newly decide the bases for their lives, including where and how they will live and what form their relationships with their children and with their former partners will take. These can seem overwhelming decisions and yet they must be made. At the same time, the parents are apt to be confused about their feelings and uncertain because of their separation of their acceptability to others. They are also often distrusting of themselves. They are, at this time, likely to be accessible to advice.

The general practitioner who becomes aware that a patient is going through separation from a partner with whom there had been a pair bond may want to explore with the patient the extent to which there is accompanying distress. If no children are involved it may be enough to reassure a distressed patient by pointing out that confused feelings that may well include intermittent feelings of desolation are normal accompaniments of separation and that such feelings subside with time. The patient might also be told that people going through separation, because their lives are so upset and because they are themselves under such emotional pressure, sometimes behave in ways they later regret. The patient

41

might be cautioned not only to try to act in a sensible fashion but also to be forgiving of his or her failures to be sensible.

It may be useful for the general practitioner to schedule a further appointment with the patient for 1 or 2 months hence, that can be cancelled by the patient if things are going well. That further appointment can demonstrate to the patient the general practitioner's continued concern and availability. At the subsequent visit the general practitioner might judge whether referral to a mental health professional is appropriate. Such a referral would be justified if confusion and despondency seemed to be becoming chronic.

When the separating couple has children the general practitioner might tell each separating parent that even though his or her children may seem resilient they are likely to be worried about themselves and about the parents and should be given caring attention. The parent should also be told that the more the two parents can manage amicably issues of parental access and of financial support the better it will be for the children. Parents may also need help, preferably from legal advisers or marital counsellors rather than doctors, to work out issues of parental access and financial support.

The single parent household

The separation of parents gives rise to single parent households and to non-custodial parents who are with their children only for periodic visits. The single parents, whether they are the mothers as in the usual arrangement or the fathers, may have full time paid employment as well as child care responsibilities. They are then liable regularly to find themselves close to overload. Under usual circumstances most single parents manage but should there be an illness in the household or difficulty at work they may come to the desperate realisation that they have *too much to do, too much to decide, and too many calls on their limited emotional reserves.* Under such circumstances they may turn to their children for help, no matter what the children's ages. Even without overload the weight of their responsibilities may have made them easily irritated or tearful and overanxious. Now they may become depressed and want to give up. Should an overwrought single parent in such circumstances telephone a general practitioner, perhaps for help with nerves, the doctor can be of great usefulness by answering the call with reassurance, sympathetic understanding, and an appointment for a longer talk. There is, however, a limit to the degree of involvement which is appropriate and general practitioners need to anticipate the dangers of being seen as indispensable. We should not delay once it is clear that referral to an appropriate mental health professional, social worker, or Relate counsellor is needed (see appendix).

Custody of the children

The parent who does not have custody of the children is likely to have to deal with feelings of loss. Grief may be so intense and painful that it causes the parent to make unreasonable attempts to regain custody or to demand unreasonable access. Inability to be with the children except at times of scheduled visits can lead to frustration and despair.

Here the doctor can help by providing the parent with the opportunity to express and work through his or her grief and by assuring the parent that devotion to the children, despite its difficulties, will be recognised and appreciated by the children. The doctor might also emphasise that the children benefit from having parents who remain cooperative despite separation, and the non-custodial parent and custodial parent should strive to maintain a cooperative relationship as best they can.

Remarriage

A new marriage or similar relationship of a divorced or separated parent is likely to be a time in which the parent is hopeful of a happy future. For that parent's children, however, it may well be a time of apprehension. The children are likely to worry about how they can reconcile their continued loyalty toward their biological parent with their new relationship with the person who is to become their step-parent. They will feel deeply connected to both their biological parents but will feel no such connection to the step-parent, no matter how nice the step-parent is. Indeed, they may resent the step-parent for taking their mother or father from them.

If the step-parent has children from a former marriage the children may worry that they will have to compete with their step-siblings for their parent's attention. They will also feel themselves required to adapt to a strange and, often, unappealing new family organisation.

The doctor can be helpful to the children—and to the parent—by encouraging the parent to listen sympathetically to the children's concerns. Listening will not make the concerns disappear; it will, however, reassure the children that they have not been deserted by the parent.

Conclusions

The doctor who encounters patients troubled by an unhappy attachment relationship or by its voluntary ending or by problems associated with bringing children into a new relationship of attachment can do a good deal that is helpful. Although a positive hopeful outlook is always valuable, whether maintained by the doctor or by the patient, the patient should not be advised to buck up and stop feeling self pity. Patients will not be able to use this advice, may blame themselves for being unable to, and will surely decide that the doctor does not take their experience seriously. Instead, the doctor should recognise the patient's perplexity and should recognise, too, that most people in the patient's situation would feel similarly. The doctor should seek to establish an alliance with the patient's efforts to do his or her best even while acknowledging that the challenges are daunting. Insofar as is possible and appropriate, the doctor should "normalise" the patient's condition by explaining it as an understandable and, indeed, typical response to situations like the patient's.

Doctors should be aware of when they can usefully offer advice and when advice is likely to be disregarded. When patients are in the middle of separation the doctor's advice, if soundly based, is likely to be accepted. Useful advice would include trying to limit the changes being made in life, being cautious in making new commitments, and being forgiving of the self for mistaken actions. For parents it is almost always good advice to maintain a cooperative relationship with the other parent and to be attentive to the children's concerns.

Advice is less likely to be useful to people whose relationships are troubled than to people in the middle of separation. The life situations of the former, although unhappy, are likely to have been as they are for some time. The unhappily married may have already considered and rejected obvious remedies. Recommendations of counselling are likely to be the most useful advice the couple can be given, but the doctor should be prepared to accept a more or less tactful refusal.

Single parents may well bring perplexities to the attention of a doctor in connection with an examination of the children or, less frequently, in a phone call made in desperation. They are likely to need support in the form of sympathetic listening and encouragement to seek occasional relief from their responsibilities. Because they are without a partner with whom to share responsibility they may rely strongly on the doctor's guidance in matters of their children's health and wellbeing. For those parents bringing children into new family situations, doctors might ask whether the parents have listened to the children's concerns.

In dealing with any emotionally troubled patient the doctor should assess the frequency and level of response that is compatible with his or her practice. Probably the doctor can provide occasional support but should not assume long term responsibility for helping with emotional or familial problems.

In general, doctors should recognise their limitations of time and training as well as their strengths as knowledgeable people committed to the patient's wellbeing. They should not assume responsibilities they cannot discharge. This means that they should not promise regular appointments that their schedules will not permit nor attempt treatments, such as long term counselling of individuals or couples, for which they lack training and experience. Instead they should maintain a list of mental health professionals whom they trust, perhaps augmented by people who work in mediation and in social assistance. They should then make referrals of patients whose conditions suggest the appropriateness of extended treatment, just as they would of any patients whose conditions required the attention of specialists.

Further reading

Dividing the Child: Social and Legal Dilemmas of Custody (Cambridge, Massachusetts: Harvard University Press, 1992), by Eleanor E Maccoby and Robert Mnookin, reports findings from a study of over a thousand divorced parents. Telephone interviews were held with each parent over the course of 3 years, and information was collected about the children's wellbeing. The book describes how the parents arranged to meet their child care responsibilities and suggests the effects on the children of different custody arrangements and different qualities of parental relationships.

In their book *Second Chances: Men, Women, and Children a Decade After Divorce* (New York: Ticknor and Fields, 1989), Judith S Wallerstein and Sandra Blakeslee report findings from a study of 60 middle class families in which the parents were divorced. The findings are based on interviews with members of the families conducted regularly over 15 years, beginning with the time of divorce. The book provides detailed information on the ways in which parental divorce affects parents and children.

In *Marital Separation* (New York: Basic Books, 1975), Robert S Weiss describes how marital separation affects the emotional and social lives of people. It is based on workshops for people whose marriages were ending.

A new book by Butler and Joyce, *Counselling Couples in Relationships: an introduction to the RELATE approach*. Chichester: Wiley, 1998, is an authoritative manual for counsellors. It has been approved by Relate, the foremost couples counselling organisation in the United Kingdom.

5 Surgery and loss of body parts

PETER MAGUIRE AND
COLIN MURRAY PARKES

The loss of body parts can have distinct but overlapping psychological consequences. These can be classified as *bodily changes*, by which we mean the alterations in the way patients, their families, and others perceive their bodies and *changes of function*, by which we mean alterations in the activities and roles which they are able to carry out. Some types of surgery affect one more than the other. Thus a unilateral mastectomy may have little influence on a woman's functional ability—she will still be able to suckle children—but the influence on her body image will usually be profound. Conversely, a gastrectomy may have little effect on the body image but necessitate a major change in the type and amount of food that a person can eat. Most types of surgery, however, affect both form and function. We start by examining a clear example of just such a loss.

Amputation of a limb

The similarities between grief at loss of a body part and grief caused by the death of a loved person have been clearly demonstrated in comparative studies by Parkes of 46 people who had undergone amputation of an arm or leg and 21 who had lost a spouse.[1] When interviewed 4 to 8 weeks later people who suffered either of these losses were preoccupied with thoughts of loss; the bereaved missing the lost person and the amputees missing the loss of physical attractiveness (loss of body image) or the occupational and other physical functions that could no longer be carried out (loss of function) or both. Many bereaved spouses as well as amputees described feeling mutilated.

47

Both groups said that they had difficulty in believing in the fact of the loss and tended to avoid reminders. Both groups reported having clear visual memories of the lost person or part, and many had a strong sense of their persisting presence. This was most pronounced in the amputees as the "phantom limb." As time passed both the phantom limb and the phantom spouse tended to dwindle in significance. In the case of the amputee the phantom limb seemed to merge with the prosthesis. In both groups returning to work was associated with improvement in emotional symptoms, but only a third of amputees were able to work full time, often because of persisting arterial disease in the unamputated limb.

Adjustment problems

Ninety per cent of all amputations today are caused by the complications of chronic disease.[2] Both before and after amputation, impairment of mobility often gives rise to depression which, in turn, reduces the patient's motivation to move and delays rehabilitation.

Like bereaved spouses, those amputees in Parkes' study who had a long standing tendency to anxiety or depression (the "sensitisers") coped less well and suffered more than others.[1] They contrasted with a group of amputees, mostly men, who showed little evidence of distress at the time of the amputation. Rigid and compulsively self reliant people, they seemed to be coping well, but 13 months later they were significantly more likely to be suffering persistent pain in their phantom limb than other amputees.[3] These compared with the "identification symptoms" reported by some bereaved people who showed little grief at the time of a loss ("avoiders") but subsequently developed pains and other symptoms which often resembled those suffered by the person who died. This suggests that the persistence of pain in a phantom limb may sometimes result from the repression or avoidance of grief at the loss.

Cancer and cancer surgery

Cancer commonly causes loss of bodily functions, damage to the body image, and threat to life itself. Fear and grief are likely consequences, and, the surgical and medical treatments for cancer are often drastic and may give rise to further losses. In a psychological sense *cancer invades families*, for many lives are likely to be affected by this illness. Members of the health care team have important parts to play in helping patients and their families to prepare for the losses that are to come and to cope with them when they arise.

People vary greatly in the degree of confidence and flexibility with which they cope with threatening situations. Several studies show that the intensity of distress after the onset of cancer is determined by such factors and by the degree to which people feel that the losses occasioned by the illness have made them different from others. This, in turn, can give rise to depression, problems of sexual adjustment, and other psychological difficulties.[4-6]

One indicator of adjustment—sexual functioning—gives an idea of the magnitude of the problem. Comparative studies are few but, the effect on sexuality is surprisingly similar in cancers as varied as Hodgkin's disease and cancers of the testis, lung, and prostate.[7,8] In both of these studies between a quarter and a third of respondents in each diagnostic group thought that they had become lastingly less attractive to their partners, and a similar proportion found that their sex drive was diminished.

Similar difficulties have been reported in women after mastectomy operations.[9-11] Although the psychological consequences of surgical mutilation can be severe, they need to be set against the anxiety that patients may feel if they fear that their cancer has not been completely removed. Thus, lumpectomy has often been advocated on the grounds that it is less psychologically traumatic than mastectomy yet, in one study it was associated with a slightly higher incidence of anxiety states and depression than mastectomy.[9] Similarly, surgical treatment for carcinoma of the cervix has been shown to give rise to rather less reduction in sexual enjoyment and activity than radiotherapy.[12] On the other hand, between a quarter and a third of those men who undergo castration by orchidectomy for cancer of the testis think that the operation has made them less attractive and less able to achieve sexual satisfaction, whereas chemical castration for carcinoma of the prostate is associated with substantial improvement in psychological state.[5]

Whether or not a person undergoes surgical treatment for cancer, chemotherapy and radiotherapy will usually be carried out with loss of hair and other physical consequences. These, in turn, are a further cause for loss of self esteem, grief, and depression.

49

Cancer of the breast

Several factors have been shown to influence the way a woman reacts to a mastectomy. These include relief that a life threatening cancer has been removed, grief at loss of attractiveness, particularly among young and sexually active women, and feelings of mutilation with associated shame and loss of self esteem.[8]

Many are dissatisfied with any prosthesis that they are offered and may attempt to avoid facing the painful reality of their loss by refusing to look at their chest wall or allowing their partners to do so. Some go to the lengths of covering mirrors, dressing and undressing in the dark, and minimising the time that they spend bathing. These activities reflect an avoidant style of coping similar to that described above. It is hardly surprising that these women tend to suffer lasting depression and loss of interest in sexuality.

Cancer of the rectum

The colostomy patient has to put up with an anus in the abdominal wall and a colostomy bag which sometimes leaks, smells, and makes embarrassing noises. Small wonder that in one study over a half the patients who underwent this operation no longer enjoyed sex, a third continued to feel dirty, embarrassed, and unclean, and a quarter (the "sensitisers") remained preoccupied with their stoma. One in six shut themselves up at home and avoided social situations.[13]

Those who are treated with abdominoperineal resection suffer more than those who have operations that retain the anal sphincter. These considerations are more important in determining psychological adjustment than the nature of the cancer.

Cancer of the female reproductive organs

Surgery of the ovary, cervix, endometrium, and vulva are associated in a quarter to a third of patients with loss of self esteem, feelings of unattractiveness, loss of femininity, and sexual or other marital problems. These are often associated with persisting anxiety and depression.

Unfortunately those treated by means of radiotherapy have similar problems. Sometimes this results from a direct physical effect, as when radiation administered per vagina causes stenosis or loss of lubrication with consequent pain on intercourse.[11] Feelings of shame or stigma are sometimes aggravated if patients attribute their cancer to promiscuity or think that others are making such attributions.[14]

Cancer of the head and neck

This type of cancer is hard to ignore or conceal. It commonly causes mutilation and loss of taste, smell, and other functions as well as being a major threat to life. It comes as no surprise that between 29%[13] and 40%[15] of patients become depressed, even before the results of biopsy are known. As with other types of bodily loss the reaction is influenced by lack of social support and other causes of vulnerability in addition to the disturbance of body image.[16]

Most patients do not want to burden their doctors and nurses or to be thought ungrateful or complaining about operations and treatments that may have saved their lives. Paradoxically, the more caring the professional staff the less likely the patients are to burden them with their problems.

Cardiac surgery

We might think that since cardiac surgery has little effect on the body image and most patients are likely to experience restoration of function rather than impairment the psychological impact would be relatively slight and might be positive rather than negative. Yet, in one study over half the elderly patients who underwent cardiac surgery suffered an adjustment disorder.[17] Why should this be?

The answer seems to lie in the special significance of the heart. This is experienced as the symbol and source of life, an internal clock that ticks our life away until it stops, dead. It follows that *any interference with the heart is likely to undermine our sense of the world as a safe place and of our body as a stronghold.* Cardiac surgery brings home to the patient the seriousness of their illness and is an understandable cause of fear. The incidence of preoperative distress correlates with its incidence after operation. Anxiety has physiological effects on the heart and these in turn may increase fear and feed into a vicious circle of fear and cardiac symptoms. In addition, open heart surgery may also give rise to some degree of cognitive impairment, particularly in elderly patients, making it more difficult for the them to cope with the emotional demands of the operation.

In these circumstances it is not surprising to find that many cardiac patients remain fearful of exerting themselves and apprehensive even when good cardiac function has been restored by surgery. This is most obvious in sexual activity and explains the occurrence of erectile disfunction and loss of desire in these patients (see the recent review by Borowitz *et al* of 35 studies[18]).

The prevention of problems

Members of the caring professions are always to hand when people suffer bodily losses. Counselling, in the form of information and advice given before surgery, emotional support, and the provision of opportunities to discuss any problems that are anticipated, reduces the prevalence of psychological problems after mastectomy[19] and cardiac surgery.[20]

If an operation is planned *the patient will need to be properly prepared for both the operation and its short term and long term consequences.* Those about to undergo an amputation should be warned that a phantom limb, which may be painful, might persist for a while and they should be invited to share any doubts or fears they have. This enables the carer to reassure them when fears are needless and to support them in grieving for the losses that are inevitable. It also increases the probability that the patient will agree to undergo the surgery. Such support has been shown to increase the probability that the patient will cope effectively with the loss.[2]

Recognition of problems after surgery

Despite the prevalence of the sexual and other problems described above, they are detected and treated in only a small minority of patients.

Patients assume that these problems are a necessary consequence of the treatment, there is nothing to be done, and there is therefore no point in disclosing them. Professional staff, on the other hand, tend to assume that if patients have problems they will disclose them. They also assume that if staff ask about a problem they will sensitise the patient and create the very problem they fear. Thus, in one study of women undergoing mastectomy, not one had been asked a direct question about how she felt about the impact of surgery.[21]

Any person who has undergone surgery or other treatment that has led to the loss of a body part or function should be asked how they feel about the loss ("How have you felt about losing your breast?") and the impact on mood, day to day life, relationships, and sexuality ("Can you look at the scar?", "Is it having any effect on your physical relationship?"). If there is evidence of mood disturbance it is important to establish whether or not this amounts to an affective disorder.

It is also important to discover how well the family are coping ("How does your partner feel about the effects of your operation?", "Can you talk to your family about their feelings?"). A man who has lost a testis or a woman who has lost a breast needs to know that their partner still finds them attractive. When surgery is carried out in childhood it is particularly important to involve parents in the support system as their attitudes and overprotective behaviour can undermine rehabilitation.

Management of problems

Despite some research which throws doubt on the lasting benefits of routine use of professional counsellors for stoma patients,[22] there can be little doubt that the kind of emotional support and information that can be given by a doctor or nurse is of great value to patients about to undergo major surgery and there is a minority of patients who will require additional help with particular problems. Other members of the patient's family, particularly spouses, whose lives are also affected by the patient's illness or disability, will also need support.

"Avoiders" may need opportunities to talk through the implications of their loss and reassurance of the normality of grief and of its physical and emotional consequences. "Sensitisers" are more likely to benefit from meeting other patients who have undergone similar surgery and can help to reassure them that it is possible to live with disabilities and to induct them into the world of the postsurgical patient.

Anything which increases mobility and enhances the patient's confidence and self esteem will facilitate both kinds of transition.[23] Well conducted postoperative exercise programmes will restore the patient's confidence in their bodies; this is particularly important after cardiac surgery when spouses, and even doctors and nurses, commonly aggravate patients' fears by treating them as if they were extremely fragile.[24] Organisations such as Cancer Link and Ostomy Clubs (for people with stomas) give newcomers opportunities to learn from veterans how to live with their disabilities (see appendix).

People with damaged bodies may have longed for the day when they will again feel strong and safe. They approach surgery with a mixture of hope and dread. *All too often their fear creates the very situation they dread.* The physical manifestations of fear (which include the effects of both hyperventilation and autonomic disturbance) are easily misinterpreted as symptoms of bodily damage. It is important for medical attendants to provide positive reassurance and explanation for all such symptoms and to avoid overinvestigation (which serves only to convince patients that their doctors are as worried as they are). Anxiety management includes techniques for muscular relaxation and imaging (envisaging relaxing scenes and situations). Anxious patients may also benefit from occasional doses of an anxiolytic drug at times of particular stress.

The fact that someone who is clinically depressed has lost a limb or a breast does not mean that they will not respond to antidepressant medication, and there is no evidence that these drugs interfere with the process of grieving. When there are clinical indications for their use they should be given in full dose and for at least 4 months.

Clinical psychologists have much to offer. Cognitive behaviour therapies challenge patients' misperceptions of themselves, and others can be very helpful when problems with body image persist. They are of particular value for disturbance of mood and sexuality associated with problems of body image.[25]

Surgical correction of disfigurement can also have a positive influence on body image, and operations such as breast reconstruction and the re-siting or modification of stomas can have profound benefits. Patients should have realistic expectations and be properly prepared.

Although many sexual problems respond to appropriate education, reassurance, and support, those that do not may be helped by conjoint sexual therapy for both patient and partner. Sometimes a recent loss may uncover sexual and other problems that go back a long way. In such cases dynamic psychotherapy may be the treatment of choice. In all of these situations the general practitioner, who is likely to be the only person in a position to give long term support, is a key figure. The special problems that arise when a fatal outcome becomes likely will be discussed in chapters 10 and 11.

Recommended reading

Although over 20 years old Howell's compilation of 36 papers on *Psychiatric Aspects of Surgery* is still a useful source of information on a wide range of issues.[26]

1 Parkes CM. Psycho-social transitions: comparison between reactions to loss of a limb and loss of a spouse. *Br J Psychiatry* 1975;**127**:204–10.

2 Butler DJ, Turkal NW, Seidl JJ. Amputation: preoperative psychological preparation. *J Am Board Fam Pract* 1975;**5**:69–73.

3 Parkes CM. Factors determining the persistence of phantom pain in the amputee. *J Psychosom Med* 1973;**17**:97–108.

4 Weisman A, Worden JW. *Coping and vulnerability in cancer patients. Research report project Omega*. Boston, Massachusetts: Harvard Medical School, 1977.

5 Parle M, Jones B, Maguire P. Maladaptive coping and affective disorders in cancer patients. *Psychol Med* 1996;**26**:735–44.

6 Harrison J, Maguire P, Ibbotson T, *et al.* Concerns, confiding and psychiatric disorder in newly diagnosed cancer patients: a descriptive study. *Psycho-Oncol* 1994;**3**:173–9.

7 Hannah MT, Gritz ER, Wellisch DK, *et al.* Changes in marital and sexual functioning in long term survivors and their spouses: testicular cancer versus Hodgkin's disease. *Psycho-Oncol* 1992;**1**:89–103.

8 Schag CAC, Ganz PA, Wing DS. *et al.* Quality of life in adult survivors of lung, colon and prostate cancers. *Qual Life Res* 1994;**3**:127–41.

9 Maguire P. Psychological aspects of surgical oncology. In: *Surgical oncology.* Veronese U, ed. Berlin: Springer Verlag, 1989:272–81.

10 Fallowfield LJ, Baum M, Maguire P. Effects of breast conservation on psychological morbidity associated with the diagnosis and treatment of early breast cancer *BMJ* 1986;**293**:1331–4.

11 Maguire P, Lee EG, Bevington DJ, *et al.* Psychiatric problems in the first year after mastectomy. *BMJ*. 1978;**i**:963–5.

12 Yeo BK, Perera I. Sexuality of women with carcinoma of the cervix. *Ann Med Singapore* 1995;**24**:676–8.

13 McDonald LD, Anderson HR. Stigma in patients with rectal cancer: a community study. *J Epidemiol Community Health* 1984;**38**:284–90.

14 Davies ADM, Davies C, Delpo MC. Depression and anxiety in patients undergoing diagnostic investigations for head and neck cancer. *Br J Psychiatry* 1986;**149**:491–3.

15 Morton RP, Davies ADM, Baker J, *et al.* Quality of life in treated head and neck cancer patients. *Clinical Otorhinolarynol* 1984;**9**:181–5.

16 Baile WF, Gilbertini M, Scott L, *et al.* Depression and tumour stage in cancer of the head and neck. *Psycho-Oncol* 1992;**1**:15–24.

17 Oxman TE, Barrett JE, Freeman DH, *et al.* Frequency and correlates of adjustment disorder related to cardiac surgery in older patients. *Psychosomatics* 1994;**35**:557–68.
18 Borowicz LM, Goldsborough MA, Selnes OA, *et al.* Neuropsychological change after cardiac surgery. *J Cardiothorac Vasc Anesth* 1996;**10**:105–11.
19 Maguire P, Tait A, Brooke M, *et al.* Effects of counselling on the psychiatric morbidity associated with mastectomy. *BMJ* 1981;**281**:1454–6.
20 Walter PJ, Mohan R, Dahan-Mizrahl S. Quality of life after open heart surgery. *Qual Life Res* 1992;**1**:77–83.
21 Maguire P, Brooke M, Tait A, *et al.* Effect of counselling on physical disability and social recovery after mastectomy. *Clin Oncol* 1983;**9**:319–24.
22 Wade BE. Colostomy patients' psychological adjustment at ten weeks and one year after surgery in districts which employed stoma care nurses and districts which did not. *J Adv Nurs* 1990;**15**:1297–304.
23 Nissen SJ, Newman WP. Factors influencing reintegration to normal living after amputation. *Arch Phys Med Rehabil* 1992;**73**:548–51.
24 Gortner SR, Jenkins LS. Self-efficacy and activity level following cardiac surgery. *J Adv Nurs* 1990;**15**:1132–8.
25 Tarrier N, Maguire P. Treatment of psychological stress following mastectomy. *Behav Res Ther* 1984;**22**:81–4.
26 Howells JG. *Modern perspectives in the psychiatric aspects of surgery.* New York: Brunner/Mazel, 1976.

6 Loss of sensory and cognitive functions

ROY FITZGERALD AND
COLIN MURRAY PARKES

Sensory and cognitive functions enable us to orient ourselves in the world, they make us aware of dangers and rewards, they mediate many sources of pleasure and of pain, and they are the means by which we receive messages from others. It follows that anything which seriously impairs sensory or cognitive function is bound to have profound psychological effects, not only on the person who suffers it but also on the family, friends, workmates, and care givers with whom the patient attempts to communicate.

Sensory and cognitive losses disable the doctor as well as the patient. When we attempt to communicate with deaf people, their deafness renders us dumb. Blindness in our patients deprives us of the ability to use non-verbal communication. An aphasic person effectively teaches us what it feels like to be deaf. The brain damaged patient makes us feel stupid. We experience the same frustration as they do and some of the same pain.

The situation is particularly hard when the circumstances demand sensitive and empathic communication, for it is this very subtlety that is most difficult to achieve. The fact that, unlike the patient, we can escape from the frustration—by escaping from the patient—encourages us to do just that. We do our duty, inform them of the help that is available to them, then leave it all to them. We give up trying to communicate, avoid interaction, and inadvertently indicate that we wish they would stop troubling us. Consequently, it is common for patients who suffer from communication defects to feel that *they have become a burden to all who meet them.* They may be tempted to give up trying to cope with a world that feels unappealing and rejecting.

Loss of sight

In this chapter we shall take blindness as our prime example. Our exploration of the reaction to blindness causes us to ask why the services that exist to help blind people often fail to enable them to achieve a satisfactory adjustment to the loss of their sight. We suggest that an understanding of the psychological reaction to blindness, in both patient and carers, can open the door to effective rehabilitation. We then move on to consider, briefly, the similar problems that arise after other types of sensory and cognitive loss.

The London study

Our examination of the problems of adjusting to blindness stems from a study by one of us of 66 adult Londoners aged 21 to 65 years who were followed up for a mean of 5.2 years after being registered as blind.[1-5] This research was supplemented by clinical studies and consultation with service providers for the blind, mainly in the United States over a period of 25 years.

The onset of blindness

Most blind people are not born blind, they become blind (by blindness we mean loss of vision of such degree that a person is no longer able to work at any job without learning the special skills that will make this possible). This means that having learned to rely on their sight to recognise and relate to the world they must radically revise their basic assumptions about the world. It is not surprising that blindness is usually an overwhelming personal and family catastrophe affecting the patient's mobility, work, personal relationships, and much else besides.

Although loss of sight is sometimes gradual, three fifths of those in the London study had less than a year between onset of symptoms and loss of useful vision, with 35% becoming blind in less than 2 weeks. Causes, in order of prevalence, included diabetic retinopathy, optic atrophies, macular degeneration, retinitis pigmentosa, myopias (including choreoretinal degeneration), retinal detachment, inflammatory processes, vascular occlusion, and glaucoma. There were no cases of loss of sight resulting from trauma, although these have been reported more frequently in military populations.

The reaction to blindness

Table 6.1 shows the prevalence of the principal psychological features which were reported when blindness was established.

Table 6.1 Prevalence of psychological reactions to blindness in 66 adults

Feature	No(%)
Recurrent affective responses to blindness	
Longing to see what cannot be seen	64 (97)
Events trigger loss of sight feelings	48 (73)
Longing for work experiences	27 (41)
Cognitive and motor responses	
Preoccupation with visual past, daydreams.	55 (83)
Eye irritation, pain, and/or headaches	44 (67)
Aware of trying to see more than able	34 (52)
Continuing sight dependent activities (for example, watching TV)	24 (36)
Using optical aids (for example, spectacles) that no longer help	17 (26)
Maladaptive coping and denial	
Persistent longing for sight	42 (64)*
Refusing help and rehabilitation for blindness	38 (58)
False belief that sight not lost	35 (53)
Avoiding other blind people	26 (39)*
Going to faith healers to restore sight	23 (35)
Unrealistic sight dependent plans	12 (18)

* Significantly correlated with poor adjustment $0.05 > P > 0.02$.

These resemble the reaction to bereavement by death and other traumatic losses.

Despite considerable individual variation the reaction tended to follow the following sequence.

Shock or disbelief

was the initial reaction to loss of sight, which did not prevent major feelings of distress. "I didn't believe it was happening to me" or "It's not permanent" were common reactions.

Pining

for what is lost was soon evident, and 97% reported longing to see those things that they could not now see. This was associated in over 70% with high anxiety and episodes of tearfulness. Parents longed to see their children grow up; others intensely missed the sight of the countryside when out walking or being able to see familiar rooms at home. These pangs of grief for the visual world were triggered by anything that forced the patient to confront the reality of blindness. For instance, a blind man described his distress when his granddaughter asked him to read a story. These experiences were intensely frustrating and evoked feelings of irritability and anger.

Depression

is an understandable reaction which followed the episodes of pining and alternated with them. It was evident in 85% of subjects and continued after the pining and accompanying tearfulness had declined.

Resolution

often followed one or more turning points when the blind person began to think of the future in a positive way and to make plans. The turning point was associated with increased self esteem and attempts at mastery reflected in self sufficient acts such as preparing meals. The depression lifted, and crying and social withdrawal diminished. As one man of 62 described it, "I don't feel depressed or wish I was dead any more. In fact, I've been going to the social club for the blind. I've never felt better, I even forget that I've lost my sight at times."

Long term adjustment

Unfortunately this progress towards recovery occurred in less than a half of the subjects studied; for the rest lasting depression and other psychological disability persisted. *Anxiety and depression persisted in a half the subjects*, and substantial minorities had a lasting decline in self esteem, sleep disturbance, and social withdrawal. A quarter reported excessive gain in weight, and a third reported episodes of irritability and anger. Persisting pain in the eyes and headache were common and often thought to be of psychogenic origin. Several young married men had lasting sexual problems, and people who increased their consumption of alcohol or tobacco seldom returned to levels of consumption before their illness.

Determinants of poor outcome

A major correlate of delayed recovery was persistent denial of blindness. Over half (53%) of patients clung to an unrealistic hope of recovery, and 58% refused to learn the skills necessary to adjusting to life as a blind person. A third had been to faith healers in the hope of recovering their sight. But it was not only faith healers who colluded with their denial, *all too often unrealistic hopes had been kept alive by doctors who, out of a reluctance to upset the patient, pretended that there was still hope of recovery,* often by arranging repeated and unnecessary examinations.

Table 6.1 shows the prevalence with which recently blind adults had persisting visual experiences. No less than 36% continued to undertake sight dependent activities and 26% continued to use optical aids which were no longer of any use to them. Of the 53 who could recall dreams, 49 continued to experience vivid visual dreams and, although these tended to diminish over time, a quarter of them did not change.

Denial of blindness correlated with depression, which seems to imply that denial is seldom a satisfactory solution to the problem of blindness; either it represents a desperate attempt to keep depression at bay by denying its cause or repeated disappointment of the hope of recovery eventually caused the patient to despair. In either case, the feeling of helplessness which regularly accompanies depression further undermined motivation and deterred efforts towards rehabilitation.

Other factors associated with poor outcome were a history of maladjustment before the illness, low educational and occupational attainment, and persisting physical ill health. A history of maladjustment is a reflection of vulnerability which, as we saw in previous chapters, is a likely predictor of difficulty in coping with stress. Low educational and work attainment may act in several ways, perhaps by giving people fewer choices, less confidence in their ability to succeed, and less money with which to purchase help.

Persisting physical ill health makes additional demands on people at a time when they are already at full stretch. Thus, 10 out of 14 people who had undergone operative surgery after going blind suffered lasting depression compared with only 12 out of 29 who had not. Patients (particularly old people) find it hard to begin the long struggle to learn blind skills when they already have other battles to fight to survive diabetes or other health problems. It is tempting for them to give up, subside into a slough of depression, and neglect themselves; this, in turn, may further undermine their health.

On the other hand, a few people had had no significant reaction to blindness. These included a woman who had been trained as a physiotherapist to work with the blind and several others who had blind relatives or had worked in one way or another with blind people. Such experience may have acted as a kind of preparation, making people aware of the fact that it is possible to cope with this disorder and by creating a realistic set of expectations. As in the case of other transitions, their possession of an accurate internal model of the world they were now entering made the adjustment much simpler.

Another factor favouring good outcome was the establishment of important relationships with care givers or with other blind people.

Preparation for and management of blindness

The foregoing study has many implications for the preparation of people who are suffering progressive blindness and the management of the problems that arise. The following measures have proved successful in clinical practice.

In the long term, patients and their families appreciate the doctor being frank about the poor prognosis and the finality of blindness. While it is always difficult to be the bearer of bad news, and especially difficult for the ophthalmologist who is dedicated to preserving sight, it has been found over and over again that it is vital to be forthright and direct but gentle and supportive with the communication of diagnosis and prognosis.

It is also important for the doctor to be quite clear about the futility of seeking multiple opinions and undertaking expensive and wasteful treatments. While it is important to support religious faith when this is present, that does not mean that we should encourage people to seek help from psychics or faith healers. Experience shows that blind people who seek for miraculous cures are doomed to disappointment.

It is usually possible to prepare people for the likelihood that they will lose their sight, and this will reduce the shock when that stage is reached. It also helps to point out to the patient the frequency with which people are tempted to deny their blindness and the likely consequences of this. In doing this we need to be aware that we are removing hope and we need to put another hope in its place—that is, our confidence in the hope of rehabilitation. *People need permission to grieve*. They need to recognise that this is a normal and natural reaction to loss and not a weakness or a sign that they are "breaking down". They need to know that their grief will eventually abate and that we will stand by them through the transition to a new adjustment to life.

Members of the family also need opportunities to share their grief as the impact of the patient's blindness on their own lives becomes apparent. They need information, support and opportunities to talk through these implications with someone who is well acquainted with the facilities that exist to help them. In fact they need to be involved in the rehabilitation process from the start so that they become *part of the rehabilitation team as well as recipients of its care*. Failure to do this may bring about the situation in which an anxious wife or husband is undermining the team's effort to help the patient to become autonomous.

Depression, as we have seen, is a common problem. Occasionally blindness will trigger a major depressive illness for which appropriate antidepressant medication is needed. Suicide, though rare, can be a danger, and we must not hesitate to question people regarding any wish to kill themselves. Psychiatric referral may be appropriate for the treatment of unremitting depression, risk of suicide, and other severe psychopathology. Occasionally brief admission to a psychiatric unit will be needed, and such units should be equipped to assist with orientation skills and training in the activities of daily living needed by blind people.

More often, depression is a reflection of the difficulties that people face in coming to terms with blindness. Proper attention to physical health and a positive attitude on the part of all the caring team is essential. It is important for a member of the primary care team to be familiar with the available network of rehabilitation services that are available to the blind and to ensure that the patient makes full use of these. If, as is often the case, agencies are slow to act, waiting lists are long, and paperwork burdensome the patient and family must be prepared for this and supported through the periods of waiting.

The ophthalmologist can help by keeping in occasional contact with the patient to ensure that his or her needs for medical, emotional, and social support are being met. When patients are being referred to a new agency it is important that the reasons for referral be made clear so that patients do not feel that they are being abandoned. A follow up interview may be indicated to check that the help that was hoped for has been given and as a guarantee that the person whom the patient has come to trust has not lost interest.

Of particular value to blind people are opportunities to meet with veterans, other blind people who have "come through the fire" and achieved a reasonable level of adjustment. Many organisations for the blind (see appendix) employ blind or partially sighted people on their staff, and there are also mutual help groups run by and for blind people. In the United Kingdom the main organisation for the blind is the Royal National Institute for the Blind (RNIB); in the United States the American Foundation for the Blind (this has branches in each state).

Group counselling has been shown to be effective,[6] and more groups should be established to help blind people to adjust to the course of blindness, support rehabilitation, monitor physical health, express feelings, review relationships inside and outside the family, and provide a microcosm in which people can explore the world that they are entering. Whenever possible these groups should be run by people who are themselves blind or partially sighted.

If, despite all our efforts, a blind person fails to meet our expectations of recovery from depression and to achieve a reasonable level of rehabilitation we should not hesitate to refer them to specialist services which combine psychiatric and psychological evaluation with rehabilitative skills. In Britain the RNIB has a rehabilitative facility in Torquay, and similar facilities are available in "centres for independent living" in many major cities.

Loss of hearing

Loss of hearing gives rise to many similar problems to those which follow loss of sight. These are dominated by fear and grief. Carers are frustrated by the difficulty in communication and commonly treat the deaf person as if he or she is stupid or wilfully deaf. *Deafness evokes less sympathy than blindness.* Fears of the deaf patient include fear of making mistakes, embarrassing others, ridicule, new situations, sudden noises, being avoided, and making oneself conspicuous.

As the disability becomes established deaf people go through the same succession of stages as described above in the lives of the newly blind—that is, from denial and disbelief, through pining and anger to retreat and depression, and, finally, if all goes well, to rehabilitation and a new adjustment.[7,8] Jack Ashley, who made a good adjustment to his own deafness, nevertheless described it as "a lifelong burden".[9]

Like blindness, deafness affects the family. One woman, whose husband did benefit from a hearing aid, described how the hearing aid, "gave me back my husband". This brings home the fact that deafness, perhaps more than blindness, "cuts you off from people". This point is also clearly illustrated by one deaf mother whose deafness was brought home to her, with particular poignancy, when she failed to hear her child fall downstairs.

Deaf people commonly take a long time to accept that there is anything wrong with their hearing and some never do. This interferes with our attempts to persuade them to learn sign language or the other skills that are needed if they are to function effectively in the world of the deaf. People with total loss of hearing often persist in attempts to use hearing aids long after these are of any value and may engage in a useless and expensive search for more effective models. *Sadly there are some professionals who collude with this denial.*

Thomas and Herbst have reported psychiatric illness in 19% and high levels of emotional disturbance in another 20% of deaf people. Much of this is associated with depression.[10] Again the implications for care are clear. People who suffer from progressive deafness need honest and accurate information, explanation, reassurance (when this is appropriate), and recognition of their right to express real grief and frustration. Their families need to be supported and to remain closely involved in the process of rehabilitation, which should be monitored to ensure that the deaf person achieves a reasonable degree of autonomy. General practitioners should provide the continuity of care that brings this about.

Aphasia

The difficulties of communicating with patients with aphasia probably explain the relative paucity of systematic studies of the psychological reaction to this condition. Even so there is strong clinical evidence which suggests that many of the problems of the aphasic patient are similar to those which have been described above. The aphasic patient's tendency to make "stupid" mistakes leads others to assume that they are indeed stupid. Consequently they may lose the respect of carers who fail to understand their needs.

Aphasic people lose their jobs and other skills, they face social isolation similar to that of the deaf person, their roles within the family undergo profound changes, and it is not surprising if they react emotionally to their predicament. Depression and feelings of worthlessness are common and sometimes amount to a "catastrophic reaction" when something happens which brings home the magnitude of their loss.[11]

Despite the common coexistence of agnosia with aphasia it is always possible to communicate with aphasic people, although this can take a long time. It is, therefore, particularly important for professionals to make available the time that is needed and not to allow our own sense of impatience to mar our relationship with the sufferer. Aphasics need to be encouraged to make full use of alternative methods of communication. Thus, one man who could not write at all carried out a long and rewarding correspondence with some children to whom he sent pictures illustrating his life. They replied in like form over several years.

When someone cannot tell us how they feel we can test out our understanding of their situation by describing how we imagine we would feel in a similar situation. The patient can usually indicate their agreement or disagreement with this insight. Most are reassured to know that we understand, even if there is no way in which we can change their situation. It is also important for them to realise that we understand that it is not they but the illness that is burdensome and that we are quite willing to share that burden.

Loss of cognitive function (confusional states, dementia, and learning disorders)

To communicate it is necessary to organise thoughts in a coherent way. This means that many of the problems of communication which we have discussed above also exist when people suffer disease in or damage to their cerebral cortex. But there are some important additional factors to be considered. *To grieve it is necessary to remember what you have lost.* This simple fact explains the relative lack of grief found in severely dementing patients. Less severe forms of brain damage may, however, give rise to great distress.

66

As long as people have sufficient mental function to remember what they have lost they can be expected to grieve; their grief, however, is likely to take different forms from that of people with intact cognition.

Acute confusional states, whatever their cause, often give rise to great distress. Anxiety itself impairs concentration and judgment, aggravating the very symptoms that caused it in the first place. The experience of disorientation can be very frightening particularly if the sufferer is in an unfamiliar environment. Well meaning nurses and doctors may be seen as strangers who are assaulting the person, and patients may hit out to defend themselves. The thought that we may be losing our mind is so frightening that it is likely to be denied. People will confabulate to explain the gaps in their memories and, because their cerebral function is impaired, these stories are often transparently ridiculous. Thus one lady who had been incontinent insisted that, "The sea came in during the night and wet my bed". Any attempt to force people to face the fact of their impairment serves only to aggravate their distress, and those who are aware that their powers are failing are acutely sensitive to ridicule or patronising behaviour.

The implications for care are clear. Whenever people are inclined to confusion we should try to maintain their orientation by providing them with reassurance and with simple and familiar cues. If they become confused at night we should turn on the light and talk in a clear and reassuring way to them. Warm and affectionate support will often produce a rapid relaxation of tension and an improvement in cognitive function. During times of lucidity it is important for the person who has been confused to know that, even if the condition should get worse again, we will continue to treat them with respect and to see them as the person they have always been. We will not treat them as a "vegetable". (*"Vegetables" are created by doctors and nurses not by illness.*) Although tranquillisers are sometimes needed to restore peace of mind, they may aggravate confusion and it is wise to keep their use to a minimum and to tail them off as soon as possible.

In the more gradually progressive forms of cognitive loss (dementia) people have time to get used to their loss of memory and are less likely to become agitated. Even so they may get upset if something forcibly brings home to them the fact of their loss of mental ability. Teasing relatives or angry staff who blame patients for being

67

"stupid" may trigger a *catastrophic reaction* in which the patient may rush off, assault people who are to hand, or burst into tears. In all such cases it is important to find out what caused the reaction so that future episodes can be prevented. While it is kind to provide people with opportunities to share their thoughts and feelings about their illness or any other losses that are troubling them we should let them set the pace. *It is unkind repeatedly to remind brain damaged people of what they have lost* in the mistaken idea that they need help to grieve. The elderly man who forgets that his wife is dead will suffer acute grief every time that a well meaning staff member brings it home to him. He may then forget what he has been told and be forced to go through the whole thing again the next day.

Although the patient's grief will usually grow less as the condition becomes worse, the same cannot be said of the *grief of the family*. It is hard for a husband or wife to accept that the sensitive, considerate and intelligent partner of 40 years has become forgetful, insensitive and incapable of the degree of abstraction necessary to see another person's point of view. Many partners and other care givers will deny the severity of the impairment and interpret the patient's behaviour as wilful or bad. It is often they, rather than the patient, who need a shoulder to cry on. Organisations such as the Alzheimer's Society (see appendix) can do much to educate carers and to provide them with mutual support. Theut *et al* gives a more extended account of the grief of the care giver.[12] (See also pp 84–5.)

The recognition that a child has a *learning disorder* can be a major cause of grief to the child's parents. They will not wish to hear and may indeed refuse to accept such a diagnosis, and the doctor must be prepared to take the time and trouble that is needed to support them through their grief.

Although the children themselves do not necessarily grieve for the loss of mental functions that they never had, they may well grieve when the reality of their difference from other children is brought home to them. This is particularly likely to happen at adolescence when they begin to feel sexually unattractive and others may even treat them as if they were a sexual menace. Those with a low mental age often enjoy playing with children younger than themselves, and this is easily misinterpreted as evidence of paedophilia. For a balanced view of these issues see Turk.[13] See also p 83 for a consideration of the needs of people with learning difficulties who suffer a bereavement.

Conclusion

Sensory defects and cognitive defects cripple the care giver as well as the patient. It is important not to treat patients as if it were they, rather than their illness, that is a burden to us. In helping people who are suffering these defects it is important for the care giver to get inside the minds of patients and their families, to understand the fears and losses that they face, to give reassurance when reassurance is possible, and to acknowledge their need to grieve when it is not. *Until people have grieved for the world that cannot be they are unlikely to be willing to accept the world that can be.* It is our role to support them through the grieving process as well as to teach them the skills that will enable them to relate to the world that they are entering.

1 Fitzgerald RG. Reactions to blindness: An exploratory study in adults with recent loss of sight, *Arch Gen Psychiatry* 1970;**22**:370–9.
2 Fitzgerald RG. Visual phenomenology in recently blind adults. *Am J Psychiatry* 1971;**127**:1533–9.
3 Fitzgerald RG. The newly blind: mental distress, somatic illness and disability. *Eye, Ear, Nose, Throat Monthly* 1973;**5**:99–101, 127–32.
4 Fitzgerald RG. Commentary on sexual behaviour in the blind. *Medical Aspects of Human Sexuality* 1973;**7**:60.
5 Fitzgerald RG, Ebert J, Chambers M. Reactions to blindness: a four year follow-up study. *Percept Mot Skills* 1987;**64**:363–78.
6 Oehler-Giarratana J, Fitzgerald RG. Group therapy with blind diabetics. *Arch Gen Psychiatry* 1980;**37**:463–7.
7 Knapp PH. Emotional aspects of hearing loss. *Psychosom Med* 1948;**10**:203–72.
8 Jones L, Kyle J, Wood P. *Words apart: losing your hearing as an adult.* London: Tavistock, 1987.
9 Ashley J. In: Orlanes H. *Adjustment to adult hearing loss.* San Diego: College Hill Press, 1985.
10 Thomas AJ, Herbst KR. Social psychological implications of acquired deafness for adults of employment age. *Br J Audiol* 1980;**14**:76–85.
11 Swash M, Oxbury J, eds. *Clinical neurology,* Vol 1. London: Churchill Livingstone, 1991.
12 Theut SK, Jordan L, Ross LA, *et al.* Caregiver's anticipatory grief in dementia. *Int J Ageing Hum Dev* 1991;**33**:113–8.
13 Turk J. Forensic aspects of mental handicap. *Br J Psychiatry* 1989;**155**:591–4.

7 Occupational loss

LEONARD FAGIN

Tom was a 38 year old scaffolder working on the Tyneside docks, married with two children. Dr Kingsley had treated him for his psoriasis in the past, with good response; fortunately it had not affected his joints. He knew Tom was of the forbearing type and not one to complain easily. Examining his elbow and scalp, he confirmed a serious exacerbation of scaly lesions.

"The psoriasis has returned with a bit of a vengeance. Had it long?"

"About 3 weeks. I was hoping it would clear up without having to come and bother you. But it's getting worse. It's not been my year."

"What do you mean?"

"I was laid off a couple of months ago. No warning, although we had an idea the company wasn't getting any orders in. No jobs on the docks these days, so things not looking too bright."

"That must be a worry."

"Aye, and its affecting all of us at home. Not just the money, which is a problem as well, it's a strain to be in the house with nothing to do. Me and the wife are arguing more than usual, and even the kids are tetchy. I'm afraid I'm smoking and drinking a bit too much too, even when I can't afford it."

Unemployment and health—epidemiological aspects

Tom was one of the men and their families we interviewed in the late 1970s at the time of massive increases in unemployment in the United Kingdom. Interestingly, his psoriasis cleared up only after he developed a back problem which forced him to take bed rest and get the full attention of his wife, who had to look after him. It was only after he secured a permanent job on an oil rig that both problems cleared up. This observation, which was seen

70

time and time again, identified "flight into ill health", a non-conscious need to justify joblessness in once proud working men through symptomatic presentation.[1]

What role does the general practitioner have when confronted with a clinical picture of this nature, where an obvious social stressor impinges on a vulnerable individual as well as his or her family? Some say that unemployment is not a medical problem, but there is little doubt that its consequences are. In this chapter I will principally cover issues relating to enforced unemployment and briefly describe aspects of loss associated with retirement.

In a recent editorial in the *Scandinavian Journal of Primary Health Care*, Steinar Westin asked: "How can we best meet the needs of the unemployed without introducing unnecessary medicalisation of their problems?".[2] Clausen and others in the same issue warned that" . . . (we) must not give the impression that doctors can solve unemployment problems. Work is the only solution".[3]

They raise this in the context of evidence from research of increases in consultation rates to primary care in the time leading up to and after unemployment. In fact there is now a wealth of reports linking the experience of unemployment to a host of health indices, including psychological and psychosomatic symptoms, suicide, and mortality.[4-11] The Office of Health Economics calculated the extra primary health care costs due to unemployment, reporting a net excess of £28 million per year on general practitioner consultations alone or a 1.2% increase on the basis of unemployment rates of 9.1%.[12] These figures did not include the costs of prescriptions and hospital services nor social security benefits. This becomes particularly important if we question the role of medical practitioners in justifying sick leave through certification, thus using health care as a controller of work discipline.[13] In England, Pringle and Morton-Jones have reported that unemployment rates are useful predictors of prescribing trends in general practice,[14] while the Jarman index of social deprivation is comparatively weak.

Caution, however, must be exercised in taking action on the basis of this reasoning. *Unemployment rates, even when accurately measured, are composite figures encompassing many different underlying individual experiences*, which include the manner in which the job was lost, previous individual or familial experiences without work, the perceived level of local unemployment, the expectation of anticipated redundancy, the inability to find a first job or to secure

71

employment after temporary voluntary withdrawal from the labour market, and other factors, all of which contribute with different weightings to the overall and specific psychological and health outcomes. Conversely, the experience of unemployment can result in other phenomena, such as the establishment of a community cohesive response or an alternative lifestyle, which can sometimes reduce the negative effects on psychological wellbeing.

While the link between psychiatric disorders and unemployment is the strongest and most researched, there is now a considerable body of evidence to associate unemployment with overall mortality[15-19] general morbidity,[20,21] cardiovascular diseases,[15,22-25] biochemical abnormalities,[26,27] vehicle accidents,[28] violence, and substance abuse.

A number of *hypotheses* have been proposed to explain how psychological and socioeconomic traumas are linked with organic symptoms; none of them are entirely satisfactory, and they remain speculative.[29] The host resistance theory assumes that stresses contribute to "psychological and physical susceptibility", although this is poorly defined.[16] The "unhealthy lifestyle" of unemployed people, in terms of increase of tobacco and alcohol consumption or poor dietary intake, may also contribute to ill health.[3] Changes in serum lipids, calcium concentrations, and blood pressure have been consistently reported in recently unemployed people and those with job insecurity,[27] and these may be components of a central pathway explaining the increase in morbidity and mortality, probably mediated through neuroendocrine transmitters.

Most of the studies have focused on unemployed men. There is still a need to explore the possible deleterious effects on jobless women, on spouses and children of unemployed people, and particularly among the young who have never had jobs.[29]

Theoretical issues

It is important to look at the theoretical framework which underpins much of this research. Many researchers do not make specific reference to such a theoretical position and often fit a perspective after they have collected data. Hammarstrom attempts to categorise the following theories underlying the association between unemployment and psychological wellbeing and health,[30] which I have attempted to refine.

The loss theory

Following Marie Jahoda's seminal studies,[31] this approach looks at the experience of unemployment as one of loss of the "latent functions" of the job, which leaves aside income reduction. These functions are:

- Imposing a time structure
- Providing regular shared experiences and contacts with others outside the family
- Linking to transcendental goals and purposes
- Defining personal status and identity
- Enforcing regular activity.

Measures of job satisfaction used in research in the field cover many of these latent functions. I believe that income loss must not be excluded from this picture as it is by definition associated with loss of lifestyle and the feeling of being able to make decisions and plan for the future (see below).

The stress theory

The effects are directly related to stressors experienced in the time leading up to job loss and after. Many potential stressors have been identified, such as heavy demands on the job leading to redundancy, concerns over an uncertain future, strained relationships at home, having to manage on a reduced income, and the sense of chronic dependency.

Learned helplessness theory

Proposed by Seligman, this theory suggests that those who have no control over their situation develop a sense of apathy, withdrawal, and eventually anxiety and depression.[32] This is particularly enhanced if the unemployed person feels personally responsible for the loss of the job. I have elsewhere described how men tend to blame themselves for their unemployment even when it was patently obvious that it was not in their control.[1]

Economic deprivation theory

In this model the primary effect of unemployment is poverty, and it is this factor which mediates between job loss and ill health and psychological malaise.

73

The loss of a job has been included with other experiences of loss with attributable psychological consequences. As in descriptions of bereavement, the emotional response to job loss has been monitored in descriptive studies, which have outlined a number of phases which are akin to the grief process. Some of the assumptions have recently been put into question.[33,34]

Archer and Rhodes' studied the *association between unemployment and grief responses*, drawing on similarities between the components of bereavement due to the loss of a significant other and other losses such as unemployment, which affect the "assumptive world", or internal representations of the world around us which have emotional and relational significance.[34–37] In a recent study they found that 16 of their sample of 60 men fulfilled the criteria for a clear grief-like response, which correlated to the degree of job attachment as well as measures of depression and anxiety. This included pining, preoccupation, and an urge to search, feelings of anger and guilt, ways of mitigating loss, and an internal loss of self worth. Like many who have studied the effects of bereavement they did not find any support for a stage theory nor did they find indications of adaptation over time to job loss in their sample; their measures were unrelated to the time since unemployment occurred. Interestingly, these measures did not show any correlation with the manner in which respondents lost their job, either through dismissal or voluntary redundancy.

Loss of self is of particular importance. Self esteem is often propped up by our achievements and activities to the point that it permits the development of an autonomous self concept, one that permits us to carry on our lives without continually having to reflect on our sense of self worth. The loss of a job and the identity that is linked to it transfers the dependency of self concept to the views of others, which are often perceived as negative and thus becomes a source of personal undermining.[38]

Other authors have also identified *variables affecting the psychological outcome after unemployment*. These include the nature and the manner in which unemployment took place, (for example, whether it was anticipated or sudden, voluntary or involuntary), the degree of attachment and personal significance of the job, the presence of negative features in the job environment, the level of familial and social support, previous experiences of job and other losses, financial security, opportunities for re-employment, and, finally, individual characteristics in terms of self esteem, intelligence, physical and mental ill health, ability to express feelings, and personal and creative internal resources.

Is loss of a job necessarily a cause for grief?

The psychological consequences of job loss do not always follow a straightforward course. Jobs impose negative pressures, such as deadlines, timetables, job overload, conflicts with peers and management, boring, repetitive, and mundane tasks, physical and mental exhaustion, restriction of broader interests and activities, and environmental stressors such as noise and air pollution. Losing a satisfying job will have different effects than losing one that is dissatisfying. Graetz in his 4 year longitudinal survey of a large sample of 16–25 year olds in Australia reported that the highest scores on Goldberg's general health questionnaire (GHQ) were in those who were in dissatisfying jobs, more so than those who remained unemployed.[39] For those who lost their jobs, GHQ scores were marginally higher in those who lost satisfying jobs, while those who had no feelings either way showed no significant differences after losing their jobs. Interestingly, those who lost dissatisfying jobs showed a minor improvement in their GHQ scores. This survey adds weight to the importance of considering job loss as a potential cause for a grief response, but what is crucial to bear in mind is the quality of the relation between what is lost and those that experience it. This also applies to those whose jobs change for the worse. What is lost is not the job but the satisfaction derived from it. In fact, one can conclude from the evidence of this study, and for this particular age group, that the quality of the job outweighs employment status in its psychological effects. School leavers and unemployed people who end up in unsatisfying jobs are no better off than their counterparts who remain on the dole. This raises the important question of investigating the circumstances and conditions of jobs that are satisfying and those that are dissatisfying as a major health initiative.

One of the potential job stressors, linked with unemployment, is job insecurity. Extended periods of job insecurity are not only predictive of job dissatisfaction but also of deleterious health outcomes, as Heaney and her colleagues reported among a group of automobile workers in the United States.[40] This particularly applies to those who have had stable jobs working in a company for many years, when the effects can be devastating (see also the paper by Joelson and Wahlquist[41]). Furthermore, unemployed people experience a reduction in social position with a component of humiliation and frustration associated with job seeking and rejection.[42]

Unemployment and the family

We must bear in mind that the effects of unemployment are not limited to the person experiencing job loss. It has been reported to extend to the spouse of the job loser, and increased rates of ischaemic heart disease have been found in the wives of unemployed men.[15] There are reports of increased wife battering and in India of women who fatally burn themselves.[43] There is weak evidence to suggest that loss of employment may be associated with child abuse.[1,44-46]

Retirement and loss

Retirement has also been described as a potential stressor, often associated with experiences of loss, but coincidental events affect this major transition in different ways. Expectations of a different lifestyle unencumbered by work pressures are not often fulfilled, and many succumb to the disappointment of restricted opportunities and the sheer boredom of winding down. This particularly affects those who have not adequately prepared in a realistic manner to the different pace of life without the structuring aspects artificially imposed by work schedules or those who have not developed alternative interests to fall back on. Increasing age and unplanned physical infirmity often dash the hopes for the future, particularly if financial problems have not been anticipated.[47] Not surprisingly retirement has been implicated as a contributory factor in depression[48] and suicide in elderly people.[49] Protracted grief reactions and pathological mourning have also been observed to surface after retirement, particularly if work was used as a "drug" to cover up previous losses, when time for reflection and loneliness allows ambivalent feelings to re-emerge.[50]

Assessment of risk

Unemployed people represent a special health risk group, but not everyone who loses a job is likely to be affected in the same way, and some will not experience stress after job loss. It is important, therefore, to distinguish those who are most likely to be adversely affected. The research reviewed above suggests that *the following are vulnerable* and need to be taken into account in assessing the risk to health of loss of employment.

- School leavers—particularly non-achievers and those isolated at school (possibility of impulsive overdoses)
- Previous history of psychosomatic or physical disability
- Young men with a dependent family
- Men and women over 50 with consistent job records and attachments to their workplace
- Those in unstable marriages or relationships
- Children of the unemployed.

These and similar issues can usually be assessed by asking a few tactful questions. Far from being upset by such questions most patients are glad of the excuse to talk about issues that are worrying them greatly. We need to bear in mind that the experience of unemployment is difficult to share, partly because it is associated with negative stigma but also because those who have been out of work for some time have often lost their ability to communicate. There is nothing to talk about.

What can the general practitioner do?

It is important to anticipate problems that may be encountered in the surgery. For those general practitioners living in areas where there is rising unemployment as a result of local redundancies, patients are likely to present themselves in the period leading up to or shortly after being informed about their redundancy.

First of all, we may need to express our sympathy and understanding of a person who is experiencing the loss of something which could have major consequences on his or her life. This is particularly relevant for those who lose their jobs unexpectedly, who have a close attachment to jobs which they have held for a considerable time, who have dependents, and who are in a financially vulnerable position and whose employment prospects are affected by age or disability.

People with a history of psychiatric illness as well as those with physical complaints which are affected by stress are likely to suffer a recurrence of their symptoms. While some of these symptoms

77

may require specific treatment it is also important to explain to the patient the connection between them and the stress associated with unemployment. It is wise to look out for symptoms of clinical depression as well as ideas of suicide, particularly in those who entirely blame themselves for their unemployment. We also need to watch for increased alcohol and tobacco consumption.

Spending a few minutes to give people the chance of sharing their feelings about their job loss may pay dividends. Sometimes the loss is experienced as so traumatic that it is difficult to speak about it at the time or it may require more focused counselling in which case it may be helpful to refer to a qualified counsellor. Other members of the family may be affected, and they may, indeed, be the first to turn up at the surgery. In such cases we will often find that one or more joint meetings is helpful. A referral to social services may be appropriate if partners or children are deemed to be at risk or if there is undue financial hardship.

Unemployment is a disempowering experience, and it is easy to understand the temptation to use ill health as an excuse for it. The main aim of intervention must be to restore the sense of dignity and identity affected by the experience and to explore with people ways in which they can resume control over their lives and not centre everything on a purely medical response to their symptoms.

Recommended reading

The Forsaken Families by Fagin and Little describes the effects of unemployment on 22 families who were studied in depth.[1] It provides rich and detailed information with important practical implications.

1 Fagin L, Little M. *The forsaken families*. London: Penguin, 1984.
2 Westin S. Does unemployment increase the use of primary health care services? *Scand J Prim Health Care* 1993;11:225–7.
3 Claussen B, Bjorndal A, Hjort PF. Health and re-employment in a two year follow up of long term unemployed. *J Epidemiol Community Health* 1993;47:14–8.
4 Beale N, Nethercott S. Job-loss and family morbidity: a study of factory closure. *J R Coll Gen Pract* 1987;35:510–4.
5 Beale N, Nethercott S. The health of industrial employees four years after redundancy. *J R Coll Gen Pract* 1987;38:390–4.
6 Claussen B. A clinical follow-up of unemployed. I. Life-style, diagnosis, treatment and reemployment. *Scand J Prim Health Care* 1993;11:211–8.

7 Claussen B. A clinical follow-up of unemployed. II. Sociomedical evaluations as predictors of re-employment. *Scand J Prim Health Care* 1993;**11**:234–40.

8 Iversen L, Sabroe S. Psychological well-being among unemployed and employed people after a company closedown: a longitudinal study. *J Social Issues* 1988; **44**:141–52.

9 Westin S, Norum D, Schlesselman JJ. Medical consequences of a factory closure: illness and disability in a four-year follow-up. *Int J Epidemiol* 1988;**17**:153–61.

10 Westin S, Schlesselman JJ, Korper M. Long-term effects of a factory closure: unemployment and disability during ten years' follow-up. *J Clin Epidemiol* 1989; **42**:435–41.

11 Yuen P, Balarajan R. Unemployment and patterns of consultations with the general practitioner. *BMJ* 1989;**298**:1212–4.

12 Office of Health Economics. *The impact of unemployment on health.* London: Office of Health Economics, 1993. (Briefing No. 29).

13 Murfin D. Medical sickness certification: why not review the role of the general practitioner? *Br J Gen Pract* 1990;**40**:313–6.

14 Pringle M, Morton-Jones A. Using unemployment rates to predict prescribing trends in England. *Br J Gen Pract* 1994;**44**:53–6.

15 Moser KA, Fox AJ, Goldblatt PO, *et al.* Stress and heart disease: evidence of associations between unemployment and heart disease from the OPCS longitudinal study. *Postgrad Med J* 1986;**62**:797–9.

16 Iversen L, Andersen O, Andersen PK, *et al.* Unemployment and mortality in Denmark, 1970–80. *BMJ* 1987;**295**:879–84.

17 Martikainen PT. Unemployment and mortality among Finnish men, 1981–5. *BMJ* 1990;**301**:407–11.

18 Stefansson C. Long-term unemployment and mortality in Sweden, 1980–86. *Soc Sci Med* 1991;**4**:419–23.

19 Morris JK, Cook DG, Shaper AG. Loss of employment and mortality. *BMJ* 1994;**308**:1135–9.

20 Cook DG, Cummins RO, Bartley MJ, *et al.* Health of unemployed middle aged men in Great Britain. *Lancet* 1982;**i**:1290–4.

21 Klein-Hesselink DJ, Spruit IP. The contribution of unemployment to socio-economic health differences. *Int J Epidemiol* 1992;**21**:329–37.

22 Franks PJ, Adamson C, Bulpitt PF, *et al.* Stroke death and unemployment in London. *J Epidemiol Community Health* 1991;**45**:16–8.

23 Janlert U, Asplund K, Weinehall L. Unemployment and cardiovascular risk indicators. *Scand J Soc Med* 1991;**20**:14–8.

24 Janlert U. Unemployment and blood pressure in Swedish building labourers. *J Intern Med* 1992;**231**:241–6.

25 Brackbill RM, Siegel PZ, Ackermann SP. Self reported hypertension among unemployed people in the United States. *BMJ* 1995;**310**:568.

26 Kasl SV, Cobb S, Brooks GW. Changes in serum uric acid and cholesterol levels in men undergoing job loss. *JAMA* 1968;**206**:1500–7.

27 Mattiasson I, Lindgarde F, Nilsson JA, *et al.* Threat of unemployment and cardiovascular risk factors: longitudinal study of quality of sleep and serum cholesterol concentrations in men threatened with redundancy. *BMJ* 1990;**301**: 461–6.

28 Partyka SC. Simple models of fatality trends revisited seven years later. *Accid Anal Prev* 1991;**23**:423–30.

29 Bethwaite P, Baker M, Pearce N, *et al.* Unemployment and the public health. *N Z Med J* 1990;**103**:48–9.

30 Hammarstrom A. Health consequences of youth unemployment—review from a gender perspective. *Soc Sci Med* 1994;**38**:699–709.

31 Jahoda M. The impact of unemployment in the 1930s and the 1970s. *Bull Br Psychol Soc* 1979;**32**:309–14.
32 Seligman MEP. *Helplessness*. San Francisco: Freeman, 1975.
33 Fryer D. Stages in the psychological response to unemployment: a (dis)integrative review article. *Curr Psychol Res Rev* 1985;**4**:257–73.
34 Archer J, Rhodes V. Bereavement and reactions to job loss: a comparative review. *Br J Social Psychol* 1987;**26**:211–24.
35 Parkes CM. Psychosocial transitions: a field for study. *Soc Sci Med* 1971;**15**: 101–15.
36 Eisenberg P, Lazarsfeld PF. The psychological effects of unemployment. *Psychol Bull* 1938;**35**:358–90.
37 Archer J, Rhodes V. The grief process and job loss. A cross sectional study. *Br J Psychol* 1993;**84**:395–410.
38 Oatley K, Bolton W. A social-cognitive theory of depression in reaction to life events. *Psychol Rev* 1985;**92**:372–88.
39 Graetz B. Health consequences of employment and unemployment: longitudinal evidence for young men and women. *Soc Sci Med* 1993;**36**:715–24.
40 Heaney C, Israel B, House J. Chronic job insecurity among automobile workers: effects on job satisfaction and health. *Soc Sci Med* 1994;**38**:1431–7.
41 Joelson L, Wahlquist L. The psychological meaning of job insecurity and job loss: results of a longitudinal study. *Soc Sci Med* 1987;**25**:179–82.
42 Ensminger ME, Celentano DD. Unemployment and psychiatric distress: social resources and coping. *Soc Sci Med* 1988;**27**:239–47.
43 Gupta RK, Svrivastava AK. Study of fatal burns cases in Kanpur (India). *Forensic Sci Int* 1987;**37**:81–9.
44 Penkower L, Bromet E, Dew M. Husbands' layoff and wives' mental health: a prospective analysis. *Arch Gen Psychiatry* 1988;**45**:994–1000.
45 Krugman R, Lenherr M, Betz L, *et al* The relationship between unemployment and physical abuse of children. *Child Abuse Negl* 1986;**10**:415–8.
46 Taitz L, King J, Nicholson J, *et al.* Unemployment and child abuse. *BMJ* 1987; **298**:1074–6.
47 Rowen R, Wilks S. Pre-retirement planning, a quality of life issue for retirement. *Employee Assistance Quarterly* 1987;**2**:45–56.
48 Muller-Spahn F, Hock C. Clinical presentation of depression in the elderly. *Geront,* 1994;**40(suppl 1)**:10–4.
49 Kirsling R. Review of suicide among elderly patients. *Psychol Reports* 1986;**59**: 359–66.
50 Paulley JW. Pathological mourning: a key factor in the psychopathogenesis of autoimmune disorders: a special contribution. *Psychoth Psychosom Year* **40**: 181–90.

8 Grief that is overlooked, hidden, or discouraged

COLIN MURRAY PARKES

In this chapter I will consider some types of loss and grief which are hidden from view, ignored, overlooked, or avoided by those who can normally be counted on to give their support. Doka has termed the effects of these "disenfranchised grief".[1]

People in this group are of particular importance to members of the health care professions for three reasons: their physical and mental health may be at risk, they seldom come to the notice of the usual caring agencies, and we often find out about them because of our access to confidential information that is hidden from others. *In fact we may be the only people who are in a position to help.*

Box 8.1 Why loss may go unrecognised

- Hidden losses associated with shame or stigma—for example, HIV infection or mental illness
- Concealment or misrepresentation of losses by care givers as when care givers conceal information from their charges—for example, children or elderly, people
- Gradual losses as when the imperceptible progression of an illness is ignored—for example, in infertility or Alzheimer's disease
- Avoided grief as when people deny their need to grieve for social or other reasons—for example, in "macho" men after any loss or mothers who have mixed feelings on the birth of a baby

---

Likely reasons are listed in box 8.1. It is not unusual for more than one of these reasons to apply.

Hidden losses

These arise when a relationship has been kept secret, when the ending of the relationship cannot be acknowledged, or when the loss is associated with feelings of shame or inadequacy. Maybe the bereaved has had a homosexual relationship that has been concealed, the death of the partner may then be a great cause for grief which the survivor may not feel free to express or share. Often *the existence of a concealed relationship has been known or guessed at by others, who collude by pretending that the relationship did not exist.* When loss occurs it is not admitted to by anyone; the bereaved try hard to hide any expression of grief for fear that their secret will be discovered and others are debarred from expressing sympathy or support.

Problems of this kind are particularly common among people with HIV infection and other diseases which may be sexually transmitted. They are also common consequences of mental illnesses, which may then be aggravated as a result.

There is a lot of truth in the saying, "To understand is to forgive" and this applies to the patient as well as the doctor. People with secrets are often trying to hide from themselves as well as from us—"If I don't tell anyone about it I won't have to think about it and can pretend that it is not true". Like most forms of denial this device is seldom successful if only because to *stop ourselves from thinking about something we have to think about it*; we have to be on our guard against the danger that we are trying to avoid. Consequently the danger is always lurking "at the back of our minds". Once the secret has been shared we no longer need to be on our guard against it.

Trust has to be earned; we have no right to expect our patients to trust us and often have to deal with this problem before attempting to deal more directly with the secrets. By reassuring the patient that anything they tell us will be treated as confidential and putting our case notes aside when confidential issues are touched on we show sensitivity and earn trust. In the end, however, it is more likely to be our non-verbal messages rather than anything we say that indicates to people that they can trust us; the welcoming smile, a hand on the shoulder at the right moment, a flash of eye contact when some particularly dangerous topic has been touched on.

Members of the health care team are often in possession of confidential information; this may make us the only people who can give support to patients with such diseases. Some sufferers will shut themselves up at home, refuse necessary treatments, and resist attempts at rehabilitation. If we criticise or browbeat them we shall only increase their feelings of insecurity and fear. If, on the other hand, we treat them with respect, withhold judgment, and encourage them to believe in themselves, we stand a much better chance of helping.

Concealment or misrepresentation of losses by care givers

Losses are often concealed or misrepresented out of kindness. A mother may not tell her 5-year old son that his father is dying because she wants to protect him from the pain that he will experience if he learns the truth. A nurse in a residential home for the elderly may not invite residents to attend the funeral of another resident because she thinks it will upset them. A doctor may give quite unjustified reassurance to a patient with heart disease for fear that the truth will cause the patient to drop dead.

In an important recent study 50 people with *learning disorders* who were being cared for in the community and who had recently lost a parent were compared with 50 others who had not been bereaved.[2] Bereaved patients were unlikely to have been warned of the coming death of their parent and unlikely to have been taken to visit the grave, and only a half of them were known to have attended the funeral. They were found to have much higher scores on a number of measures of anxiety, depression, hyperactivity, stereotyped movements, and other indicators of distress. Despite this most of the professional and family carers who looked after them were quite *unaware of their distress* and inclined to attribute their symptoms to brain damage rather than to bereavement and its secondary consequences.

Concealment of a loss often leads to bad consequences; the loss may eventually become obvious and the deception may be seen through, inaccurate information may leave the recipient ill prepared to deal with subsequent events, and an opportunity to help someone to cope with reality may have been missed. *The supposed harmful consequences of revealing the truth rarely match the harmful consequences of concealment.*

The general conclusion would seem to be that such concealment in usually a bad thing, but we should beware of being too rigid. There are some exceptions. For example, it may be wiser to delay telling a patient who is severely injured that his wife and child were killed in the same accident until he is strong enough to take the news.

Gradual losses

It is difficult to deny the fact of a major loss with which we are suddenly brought face to face; when, however, the loss is very gradual or imperceptible or people have been born with a disfigurement or disability of which they only gradually become aware, they often succeed in ignoring or minimising the implications of the loss. So too do their family, friends, and care givers, who may not understand that *depression or other psychological symptoms are often indications that they are becoming aware of their loss* and that the time has come for someone to acknowledge their need to grieve and to support them through their grief.

The *infertile couple* often deny for many years that they will never succeed in conceiving. As Bryan and Higgins put it, "Some secretly carry on hoping against all odds, if only to postpone the inevitable pain and misery of giving up hope".[3] They may not realise that their increasing irritability, their resentment of women who have had an abortion, and their loss of sexual libido are all symptoms of grief. When, eventually, they do acknowledge the true situation each partner will grieve in his or her own way and this may make it hard for them to support each other. Each may blame the other, for *infertility is always assumed to be somebody's "fault"*. Not only is infertility inconspicuous it is also something about which people often feel ashamed. Infertile couples often keep their sadness to themselves and social support from friends and family is lacking. Those unable to conceive may feel jealous of those who can and friends with children may not like to draw attention to their good fortune by sympathising.

In like manner *the wife of a man with Alzheimer's disease* may be reluctant to acknowledge that the husband she is married to is no longer the man she married. Both social pressures from her family and her allegiance to her husband force her to pretend that the gross change in his personality that has resulted from the disease has not impaired her relationship with him. Sadly her failure to acknowledge the truth may cause her to blame her spouse for failing to be the sensitive, intelligent person he always was. She may need support and understanding if she is to grieve for this real loss and find a way of living with and supporting the different spouse whom she now has. When, eventually, he dies her natural relief may make it hard for her to grieve at a time when everyone else seems to expect her to do so. (Elizabeth Forsythe gives a vivid account of a spouse's grief in her book, *Alzheimer's Disease: the Long Bereavement.*[4])

In these cases the understanding and support of members of the health care team can facilitate grieving, mitigate the feelings of anger and guilt that are inevitably present, and point the person towards the help of others who have experienced similar difficulties—for example, Issue (formerly the National Association for the Childless) and the Alzheimer's Disease Society (see appendix for further details).

Avoidance of grief

Although most people oscillate between confronting and avoiding grief, extreme avoidance of grief always takes place for a reason. People may avoid grief because they are members of a family or a society in which grief is frowned on, they may avoid it because they fear the consequences if they should express it, or they may simply believe that they have more important things to do.

Cultural influences have a strong effect on when and how grief is expressed, and anthropologists have reported great variation from one society to another (see Rosenblatt *et al* for a review of this extensive literature[5]). Whether or not the societal inhibition of grief within a culture is harmful or not is a matter for debate and research. One thing seems clear, however, we interfere with the cultures of others at our peril and should avoid applying the norms of our own culture to them. *We must respect the rights of others to mourn in their own ways.*

Even within cultures there is great variation, and *men, in particular, are often expected to inhibit their grief.* This may explain the finding that whereas women usually show more overt distress in the first year after bereavement than men and are more likely to seek psychiatric help, men take longer to return to the levels of adjustment of married controls than women.[6] They also suffer a greater increase in mortality from heart disease after bereavement than women of the same age (Jacobs reviews this literature[7]). It seems that it is the inhibition of grief that is damaging to the heart rather than its expression. Furthermore Schut *et al* have shown that *it is bereaved men, rather than women, who benefit most from therapies which encourage them to express feelings* whereas bereaved women are more likely to benefit from help in reviewing and reshaping their assumptions about the world.[8]

Cultural pressures also prescribe when and whether grief is an appropriate response. *New mothers are under considerable social pressure to rejoice rather than grieve.* For many mothers to be, however, pregnancy is unwanted, and even those who have planned for and eagerly anticipated this event may need to grieve for the many losses that result from it. Kumar and Robson found that 10% of mothers suffered clinical levels of depression during pregnancy and 14% in the first 3 months thereafter.[9] Similar figures have been reported in five other studies reviewed by Brockington.[10]

A mother may experience considerable shame if, because of feelings of depression, fear, or grief, she is *lacking in maternal feelings* for a newborn child. She is likely to be acutely conscious of the danger which her lack of feeling constitutes to her child. If she finds the courage to admit this to us we need to recognise the seriousness of the situation and to reassure her that it is not her fault (a mother cannot choose whether or not to love her child). If we help her through the period of emotional turmoil maternal feelings will usually emerge. If they do not the mother will need and should benefit from the help of a child psychologist.

Another group who tend to deny their own needs to grieve are *members of the caring professions*, particularly doctors, who spend their lives caring for others but *who often find it difficult to acknowledge their own emotional needs*. If we accept that it is appropriate and therapeutic for our patients and their families to express grief, why should we deny ourselves that privilege? It would seem that, like soldiers and members of the emergency services, we are trained to remain calm in the face of danger. This leads us to the assumption that, even when the emergency is over, we have no need to get upset. Yet such stoicism is bought at a cost, and doctors who find ways to meet their own needs for emotional expression and support are likely to become better doctors and to find greater satisfaction in their work.

Implications for care

It is difficult enough for us to cope with the endless stream of problems which our patients bring to us without having to ferret out their hidden griefs or even to find time to acknowledge our own. It seems easier to wait for crises to arise and to assume that "least said, soonest mended".

Seductive though this policy may be it is clear from the foregoing chapter that it is short sighted. *Problems that are ignored seldom go away*, they fester on, and by the time they come to our notice they may be so serious and entrenched that there is little we can do about them.

Time spent in creating the secure place in which people feel safe enough to talk about the unsafe thoughts and feelings that they are experiencing is likely to prevent further problems and *may well save time in the long run*. By indicating that we are sensitively aware of the griefs that are unspoken we tacitly give permission for people to share those griefs. One way to do this is to wait until the presenting problem has been dealt with and then ask, "Is there anything else you would like to raise?". This makes it clear that we have the time and the interest to go further. It can also help to ask about feelings; "How do you feel about that?" indicates that people do not need to be ashamed of their feelings or embarrassed to reveal them. Alternatively, we may choose to be a little more direct, "I can't help thinking that if I were in your situation I would feel very angry (or sad)". This reveals our empathy and gives implicit permission to share. Even if our guess is wrong we will have shown interest and given the person a chance to correct our mistake.

Of course, people may not open up, and we should not force the pace. We must respect their defences. In such circumstances it is worth asking ourselves if there is anybody else who might be seen as "safe". People have many *prejudices*, some will not confide in a doctor but will happily talk to a nurse, others will confide in a man but not a woman, yet others will open up only to people from a similar background or with similar problems to themselves. Much of the success of self help (or mutual help) groups stems from the feeling that, "Only people in the same boat can truly understand how I feel" (see appendix for further details).

If, despite all these alternatives, we get nowhere we may have no alternative but to bide our time. This can be very hard for *there is no one more difficult to help than the person who will not accept help*.

A couple consulted their general practitioner for help with a marital problem. The wife acknowledged that she was sexually frigid but made it clear that she was not willing to allow the doctor to probe into the possible roots of this. The doctor referred the couple to a psychologist whose behavioural methods were successful. Five years were to pass before the wife returned, on her own, to see the same general practitioner. She now wanted to talk about the sexual abuse which she had undergone from her father throughout her childhood. She later admitted that she bitterly regretted having been unable to pluck up courage to talk about these experiences at the time of her previous visits. It was only when she saw another abused woman talking on television about her experience that she realised that this was a permissible thing to do.

We shall not, of course, always succeed in our aim of helping people through these turning points in their lives and will sometimes be forced to watch helplessly while they create unnecessary suffering for themselves and others. When this happens we may need to remind ourselves that we should not expect to be omnipotent; we should share our frustration and grief with a colleague and remember the successes which, in the long run, outweigh our failures.

Recommended reading

Kenneth Doka[1] has edited a series of essays covering, in more detail, these and other types of "disenfranchised" grief.

1 Doka K, ed. *Disenfranchised grief.* Lexington, Massachusetts: Lexington Books: 1989.
2 Hollins S, Esterhuizen A. Bereavement and grief in adults with learning disabilities. *Br J Psychiatry* 1997;**170**:497–501.
3 Bryan E, Higgins R. *Infertility: new choices, new dilemmas.* Harmondsworth; Penguin, 1995.
4 Forsythe E. *Alzheimer's disease: the long bereavement.* London: Faber, 1990.
5 Rosenblatt PC, Walsh RP, Jackson DA. *Grief and mourning in cross-cultural perspective,* Washington, DC: HRAF Press, 1976.
6 Parkes CM, Weiss RS. *Recovery from bereavement.* New York: Basic Books, 1983.
7 Jacobs S. *Pathologic grief: maladaptation to loss.* Washington, DC: American Psychiatric Press, 1993.

8 Schut HAW, Stroebe M, Bout J, *et al.* Intervention for the bereaved: gender differences in the efficacy of two counselling programs. *Br J Clin Psychol* 1997; 36:63–72.
9 Kumar R, Robson KM. A prospective study of emotional disorders in childbearing women. *Br J Psychiatry* 1984;144:35.
10 Brockington I. Puerperal mental illness. *Practical Reviews in Psychiatry* 1986;8: 3–5 and 9:1–8.

9 Loss in later life

BRICE PITT

What's to lose?

It is possible to view old age as a succession of losses, gradual or sudden.[1] Stopping work means a loss of the working role, the companionship of fellow workers, a full structured day, a reduction in income, and, for those who live with another (a cynical view!), less time apart. Some people feel much diminished by retirement, hardly know what to do with themselves, and suffer a loss of status; it cannot be said that most developed societies do much to enhance the image of "senior citizens", who are liable to be patronised, marginalised or simply ignored, and part of a problem for an overburdened and underresourced welfare state.

There is a view, though, that successful ageing means compensating for some losses by making the best of change.[3] So the strains of having to commute, of living for the job, of coping with tensions, and of struggling to keep up are also lost; some pensions are at least adequate, and there are a number of concessions and allowances which make life a little cheaper for the over 60s. Having more time to oneself for one's hobbies and interests and with one's partner are often regarded as benefits. Though usually a sudden event, retirement is (unless there is unheralded redundancy) expected, and there is time to prepare for it.

Sensory loss afflicts most people as they age.[3] Presbyopia is readily remedied by glasses, presbyacusis less readily (or, perhaps, less acceptably) by hearing aids. These are very gradual processes, usually accepted without distress, though blindness or severe deafness are a different matter. The loss of teeth, with its effects on nutrition, articulation, and appearance, is far from trivial. Dental care is one of the first casualties of self neglect.

Some memory loss may be normal with the loss of neurones and neurotransmitters with ageing, though speed seems to be affected more than secondary memory and verbal IQ is very well preserved.[4] "Benign" memory impairment[5] presents no serious problems apart from the fear of dementia. In 20% of those over 80, however, that fear is, unfortunately, realised.[6]

It is not often acknowledged, except as a rueful and ribald joke, that *loss of sexual enjoyment is common and distressing and not an inevitable part of ageing*;[7] hormone replacement therapy and prostaglandins may do much to restore sexual function and enjoyment, but some older people are too shy or ashamed to seek help, fearing that they should be "past it", and may be regarded as ridiculous or "a dirty old man (or woman)".

The risk of serious health problems—stroke, myocardial infarction, heart failure, falls and fractures, arthritis, obstructive airways disease, cancer—increases with ageing,[8] though many old people are spared serious infirmity until a short final illness. Those who are less fortunate suffer loss of comfort, mobility, and life expectancy. There is a risk of widowing, especially for women, which, though perhaps less grievous for older than younger people ("The comfortable state of widowhood", remarked Mrs Peachum in *the Beggar's Opera* "Is the only hope which keeps up a wife's spirits!") still represents a major loss after 40 years or more of being together.[9]

Secondary to health problems (which make it difficult to get out and about), to reduced means (for transport and entertainment) and to the dying off of friends and family is isolation which may be accompanied by loneliness. About *half of octogenarians in the United Kingdom live alone*,[10] and the extended family is stretched thin by distance and relatively small numbers of children. Another secondary consequence of ill health, and most painful of all for many, is loss of independence. ("Do not go gentle into that good night/Rage, rage against the dying of the light!", Dylan Thomas urged his father.)

Since long term care has become ever more arbitrarily and capriciously available from the NHS, property owning old people fear loss of estate. The desire to pass on the fruits of labour, success, sound investment, or good fortune to one's family is fundamental, and the power to do so may increase an older person's self esteem. Thus the costs of continuing care add to the problems of infirmity.

Reduced life expectancy is related to age and sickness. Through life a sense of immortality gives place to the shocking awareness of inevitable death, rapidly replaced (except in time of war, epidemic, or other crisis) by a feeling that it's a long time off or denial. "Mid-life" birthdays like the 40th or 50th may precipitate fears of finality and an anxious review of achievements and ebbing potential as the "sands run out," occasionally enacted as the "mid-life crisis".[11] It is said that for some these sands run ever faster with ageing. The years get shorter, the seasons flash by, the end is nigh—but still denial is a powerful buffer. Old people make long term plans and refer to peers as "old" but not themselves. Religion, incidentally, offers fewer people the comforting prospect of an afterlife than previous generations.

A new concern, as euthanasia becomes less theoretical and more real (as already in Holland and, soon, the Northern Territory of Australia[12,13]), may be overlong survival, where life drags on without quality and the burden of infirmity falls on the family. While euthanasia may seem a boon to some it could be felt to be a duty by others, to stop being a drag on the family's emotional and financial resources.

Loss and depression

With so many vicissitudes it might be expected that the morbidity from depression in later life would be high. The evidence, however, is inconsistent and contradictory. While suicide rates peak in old age (for women in their late 60s, men around 80[14,15]) the epidemiological catchment area study in the United States found much lower rates of depression in older than in younger people.[16] Using the diagnostic interview schedule (DIS) from the diagnostic and statistical manual of the American Psychiatric Association, 3rd edition (DSM-III[17]) to diagnose major depression and dysthymic disorder the epidemiologists found a prevalence of 2–3% in those over 65—a fifth of the rate in young adults.

It has been suggested that the diagnostic interview schedule may not be a suitable instrument for the diagnosis of depression at all ages. The present state examination[18] was used for all ages over 16 in a survey of psychiatric disorder in general hospital inpatients in Oxford[19]: again, depression was least common in those over 70. Younger people might be more open, older people more guarded. Older people tend to somatise their emotional complaints, and these somatic symptoms might erroneously be attributed to organic disease. Possibly dementia could remove from consideration people who might otherwise have been recognised as depressed. Or the researchers might have happened on an unusually contented cohort, not necessarily representative of their forebears or successors.

The studies of psychiatric disorders in old people in New York and in London both showed a prevalence of "pervasive depression" of about 11%, which does not indicate any tendency to make the diagnosis more or less often in either country.[20] Rates as high as 17% have been recorded in the Gospel Oak studies in north London,[21] and these accord with rates found elsewhere in the United Kingdom by using instruments specially designed for older respondents—the geriatric mental state examination (GMS)[22] and its computerised form AGECAT[23] and the self care D.[24] The GMS gives levels of caseness from which it emerges that while the syndrome of depressive illness in later life is fairly common, the symptoms are far more so.[25]

Suppose that depression really is less common in older people: why?

- Depression carries a high mortality,[26] so sufferers may not survive into old age. This is consistent with the finding that depressive illness in later life is less likely to be associated with a family history than such illness earlier in life.[27]
- Today's oldest people are hardy survivors of poverty, large families, two world wars, and the era before antibiotics and the welfare state and tend therefore to be resilient.
- Possibly such benefits as central heating, television, allowances and entitlements, taken for granted by younger people, are appreciated by older people, who once lacked them and offset some of the losses; not having to work, for example, can be a great relief.
- The "disengagement" theory suggests that successful ageing involves a gradual and realistic letting go so that expected losses are met with philosophical detachment.[28] Thus widowing is acceptable as the inevitable outcome of a union "until death do us part," whereas the death of a son or daughter by accident or malignant disease is unexpected and deeply grievous.

93

The likelihood, though, is that depression is more common in later life but is frequently unrecognised. The evidence includes the following.

- There is a high rate of suicide in elderly people, already mentioned. Barraclough's classic study of suicides among elderly people on the south coast of England showed that most of those who died were likely to be suffering from depressive illness, had attended their general practitioners weeks before the act, and were being treated with tranquillisers, hypnotics, analgesics, and laxatives but not antidepressants.[29]
- The rate of first admissions for depressive illness to psychiatric units in England and Wales in both sexes, though more markedly in women, increases from middle life with every decade, falling off only in those over 85,[30]
- The general practitioners and general hospital doctors apparently fail to recognise depression in older people.[31] This lack of recognition may be due to lack of education, motivation ("drugs are likely to be toxic, counselling is hard to come by, and anyway it's hard to teach old dogs new tricks"), or the somewhat ageist assumption that to be depressed in old age is both normal and justified.[32]

Depressive illness in later life often follows a major adverse life event, like bereavement or an acute life threatening illness,[33] but the association may not always be that the loss precedes the depression: depression may cause loss. Depressed people tend not to take care of themselves and may become ill, have accidents, and die from self neglect as well as deliberate self harm.[26]

What to do about it?

Death is life's only certainty, but the prolongation of maturation into ageing some 30 or 40 years into the senium is a relatively new experience for most people, and guidelines about how to make the best of this bonus are scarce. Two hundred years ago men outlived one or more wives, who were likely to die in childbirth. Now most wives long outlive their husbands. They would not do so if they were to marry men some 5 years younger rather than is at present more usual a year or 2 older. Marriage "till death us do part" was easier to honour when it usually meant 10–15 rather than as now 40–50 years, as the high divorce rates in the more developed (and more aged) societies indicate.[34] Shortage of housing in the crowded United Kingdom, especially England, is aggravated by the need of divorcees for two dwellings where they used to live in one. The complexities of ex-marital partners' entitlement to a share of the former spouses' pensions are imminent.

A small consolation for high levels of unemployment is that many have been prepared for the problems of filling time and managing on reduced means long before retirement age. For these, as for those who are invalids because they are not fit for work, reaching that age may be a blessing. Others may benefit from preparation for retirement: classes and workshops are now provided by most large companies, trades union, and professional bodies.[35]

Health education not to smoke, to eat and drink moderately, to watch weight, and to take exercise is freely available and may be effective in those who are semiconverted. Health checks, either at set times (like the 75th birthday[36]) or opportunistic ("as you're here, Mr Jones, tell me how you're enjoying your retirement while I check your blood pressure") are a good opportunity for health education if practices wish to make them so. Pressure groups like Age Concern are quick to remind doctors of their responsibilities to their older patients. The use of an *"at risk" register*[37] of older people who have undergone recent life events—a recent move, illness, bereavement—or who are known to suffer chronic infirmity or are living alone may be a good use of finite resources. Screening for depression with, say, the geriatric depression scale[38] or BASDEC[39] is a good start to secondary prevention. A positive approach to the *treatment of depression* in old age, not ascribing despondency to "anno domini", perceiving the mood disorder underlying somatic complaints, use of antidepressants with confidence in sufficient dose and for long enough, and recognising the entitlement and likely efficacy of counselling for bereavement, marital problems, and in the context of established depression is needed; the consensus statement by the Colleges of General Practitioners and Psychiatrists in 1995 was a good beginning.[40]

Further education is available in many daytime and evening classes and the University of the Third Age. The adage *"if you don't use it, you lose it,"* frequently applied to sex may be equally relevant to intellectual functions. Societies in which the fitter older people help their less able peers and seniors need not be a utopian dream. Already churches, Tenants' Associations, Pensioners' Clubs, even the Freemasons often provide practical as well as financial

95

assistance, and a philosophy in which neighbourliness is not seen as prejudicial to the continuance and responsibilities of a welfare state offers a healthy symbiosis. Many retired people would and do like to "justify themselves by good works."

Finally, despair at the demographic time bomb[41] when there will be supposedly too many pensioners for the remaining workers to provide for them may have led governments into premature, panicky withdrawal of services. The Community Care Act in the United Kingdom aimed to contain the costs of residential care, subsidised by social security, by transferring responsibility to local government with a limited budget.[42] The consequence has been rigorous means testing, the expectation that those who have the means will contribute in part or wholly to their care and, as budgets run short, rationing of care to only those in the most dire need. This has meant the withdrawal of an NHS facility selectively from those who had the most right to expect it. Jefferys, however, has argued that *the "doomsday scenario" is fallacious*; true, there will be a substantial percentage increase in octogenarians in the next 20 years or so, but the actual increase in numbers is small.[43]

The greatest cause of distress and dependency—dementia—may not necessarily prove to be intrinsic to ageing. Already donepezil (lately licensed in the United Kingdom) provides temporary respite for 50–60% of sufferers from early Alzheimer's,[44] and it is not too fanciful to expect the huge volume and pace of research into that and other dementias to yield more fundamental and lasting remedies which will offset the morbidity associated with a still ageing population.

1 Butler RN, Lewis ML. *Aging and mental health: positive, psychosocial and biomedical approaches.* 3rd ed. St Louis: Mosby, 1982.

2 Palmore E. *Social patterns in normal aging. Findings from the Duke longitudinal study.* Durham, North Carolina: Duke University Press, 1981.

3 Martin J, Meltzer H, Elliott D. *OPCS surveys of disability in Great Britain. Report 1. The prevalence of disability among adults.* London: HMSO, 1988.

4 Lezak MD. *Neuropsychological assessment.* 2nd ed. Oxford: Oxford University Press, 1985.

5 Kral VA. Senescent forgetfulness: benign or malignant. *Can Med Assoc J* 1962; **86:**257–60.

6 Jorm AF. *Understanding senile dementia.* Sydney: Croom Helm, 1987.

7 Bretschneider JG, McCoy NL Sexual interest and behavior in normal 80- to 102-year-olds. *Arch Sex Behav* 1987;**17:**109–29.

8 Isaacs B. *The challenge of geriatric medicine*. Oxford: Oxford Medical Publications, Oxford University Press, 1992.

9 Parkes CM. *Bereavement: studies of grief in adult life*. Harmondsworth: Penguin, 1975.

10 Central Health Monitoring Unit. *Epidemiological overview series: the health of elderly people*. London: HMSO 1992.

11 Pitt B. Depression—the midlife crisis. *Geriatric Med* 1997;27:49–50.

12 Van der Maas PJ, van Delden JJM, Pijnenboorg L, *et al.* Euthanasia and other medical decisions concerning the end of life. *Lancet* 1991;338:669–74.

13 Roth M. Euthanasia and related issues of later life with special reference to Alzheimer's disease. *Br Med Bull* 1996;52:263.

14 Pritchard C. New patterns of suicide by age and gender in the United Kingdom and the Western World 1974–1992; an indicator of social change? *Soc Psychiatry Psychiatr Epidemiol* 1996;31:227–34.

15 Charatan F. Elderly in US have rising suicide risk. *BMJ*. 1996;312:144.

16 Myers JK, Weissman MM, Tischler GL, *et al.* Six-month prevalence of psychiatric disorder in three communities. *Arch Gen Psychiatry* 1984;41:959–67.

17 American Psychiatric Association. *Diagnostic and statistical manual of mental disorders*. 3rd ed. Washington, DC: APA, 1980.

18 Wing JK, Cooper JE, Sartorius N. *The measurement and classification of psychiatric symptoms*. Cambridge: Cambridge University Press, 1974.

19 Feldman E, Mayou R, Hawton K, *et al.* Psychiatric disorders in medical in-patients. *Q J Med* 1987;240:301–8.

20 Gurland B, Copeland JRM, Kuriansky J, *et al.* The mind and mood of ageing: mental health problems of the community elderly in New York and London. London: Croom Helm, 1983.

21 Livingston G, Hawkins A, Graham N, *et al.* The Gospel Oak study: prevalence rates of cognitive impairment, depression and activity limitation among elderly residents in inner London. *Psychol Med* 1990;20:137–46.

22 Copeland JRM, Kelleher MJ, Kellett JM, *et al.* A semi-structured clinical interview for the assessment of diagnosis and mental state in the elderly. The geriatric mental state schedule I: development and reliability. *Psychol Med* 1976; 6:439–49.

23 Copeland JRM, Dewey M, Wood N, *et al.* Range of mental illness among the elderly in the community. Prevalence in Liverpool using the GMS-AGECAT package. *Br J Psychiatry* 1987;150:815–23.

24 Bird AS, Macdonald AJD, Mann AH, *et al.* Preliminary experience with the SELF-CARE D. *Int J Geriatric Psychiatry* 1987;2:31–8.

25 Copeland JRM. What is a case, a case for what? In: King JR, Bebbington P, Robbins LN, eds. *What is a case? The problems of definition in psychiatric community surveys*. London: Grant McIntyre, 1981.

26 Murphy E, Smith R, Lindesay J, *et al.* Increased mortality rates in late-life depression. *Br J Psychiatry* 1988;152:347–53.

27 Brodaty H, Peters K, Boyce P, *et al.* Age and depression. *J Affect Dis* 1991;23: 137–49.

28 Cumming EH, Henry WE. *Growing old: The process of disengagement*. New York: Basic Books, 1961.

29 Barraclough BM. Suicide in the elderly. In: Kay DWH, Walk A, eds. *Recent developments in psychogeriatrics*. Ashford: Headley Bros, 1971:87–97.

30 Department of Health and Social Security. *In-patient statistics from the mental health enquiry for England and Wales, 1982*. London: HMSO, 1985.

31 Iliffe S, Haines A, Gallivan S, *et al.* Assessment of elderly people in general practice I. Social circumstances and mental state. *Br J Gen Pract* 1991;41:9–12.

32 Pitt B. Depressed and physically ill: how to diagnose and what to do? *Curr Opinion Psychiatry* 1995;**8**:235–6.
33 Murphy E. Social origins of depression in old age. *Br J Psychiatry* 1982;**141**: 135–42.
34 Wicks M, Henwood M. The demographic and social circumstances of elderly people. In: Gearing B, Johnson M, Heller T, eds. *Mental health problems in old age*. Chichester: Wiley, 1988.
35 Hall P. Retirement. In: Shukla RB, Brooks D, eds. *A guide to care of the elderly*. London: HMSO, 1996.
36 Williams EI. *Over 75: care, assessment and health promotion*. Oxford: Radcliffe Medical Press, 1992.
37 German PS, Shapiro S, Skinner EA, *et al*. Detection and management of mental health problems of older patients by primary care providers. *JAMA* 1987;**257**: 489–93.
38 Yesavage JA, Brink TL, Rose TL, *et al*. Development and validation of a geriatric depression scale: a preliminary report. *J Psychiatric Res* 1982;**17**:37–49.
39 Adshead F, Day Cody D, Pitt B. BASDEC: a novel screening instrument for depression in elderly medical patients. *BMJ* 1992;**305**:397.
40 Katona CE, Freeling P. Recognition and management of depression in late life in general practice. *Primary Care Psychiatry* 1995;**1**:107–13.
41 Central Statistical Office. *Annual abstract of statistics*. London: HMSO, 1994.
42 Secretaries of State for Health, Social Security, Wales and Scotland. *Caring for people*. London: HMSO, 1989. (Cm 849.) 1989.
43 Jefferys M. An ageing Britain—what is its future? In: Gearing B, Johnson M, Heller T, eds. *Mental health problems in old age*. Chichester: Wiley, 1988.
44 Kelly C, Harvey R, Cayton H. Drug treatments for Alzheimer's disease. *BMJ* 1997;**314**:693–4.

10 The dying adult

COLIN MURRAY PARKES

In this chapter I shall focus on two common problems that arise when people come close to death: fear and grief. Fear is the psychological reaction to danger, grief the reaction to the numerous losses that are likely to occur in the course of an illness that is approaching a fatal outcome. Both can be expected to arise in patients, their families, and, though we are reluctant to admit it, their doctors and other carers. Both fear and grief need to be taken into account if we are to mitigate the psychological pains of dying.

Fear

While it may seem obvious that those who are dying are likely to be afraid we should not assume that we know what they fear.

Box 10.1 Causes of fear in people with life threatening illness[1]

- Fear of separation from loved people/homes/jobs, etc.
- Fear of becoming a burden to others
- Fear of losing control
- Fear for dependents
- Fear of worsening symptoms
- Fear of being unable to complete life tasks/responsibilities
- Fear of dying
- Fear of being dead
- Fear of the fears of others (reflected fear)

Box 10.1 shows the fears, in approximate order of frequency, expressed to me as a liaison psychiatrist by patients in a hospice ward.[1] It is clear that *fears of death itself come quite far down on the list*. Fears of separation from families, being a burden, being unable to cope (letting the side down) and fears for the future of ones family and fears of pain or other symptoms of illness were all expressed more frequently. Even when people expressed a fear of dying they often made a distinction between dying and being dead. *It was the approach to death that they feared rather than the fact of being dead.*

Difficult to quantify but of particular importance is *reflected fear*, the fear which people see in the eyes of those around them or hear in the questions that are not asked; "You know, you're the first doctor to invite questions!" said one patient who had rightly concluded that if his doctors did not invite questions it must be because they were afraid of giving answers.

It follows that if we are to help people with their fears we should find out who is afraid and what their fears are. Finding out may not be easy if people are afraid to share their fears in case we make them worse. Many problems in communication arise out of fear, and *people may be afraid to talk about their fears for fear of having them confirmed*—"Doctor, Doctor, shall I die? Yes, my dear, and so shall I" (Skipping rhyme). We may need to take time to create trust and a safe place in which people can begin to talk about the things that make them feel unsafe.

Few people in our society know how people die. Their *image of death* comes from horror comics, dramatic representations in the media, and the scare stories that get passed around a family when someone dies a painful death. To most people a little illness is bad, as the illness progresses they expect the symptoms to get worse, and it is logical to expect that, at the moment of death, every symptom will be as dreadful as it can be. This image of death as the peak of suffering bears little resemblance to the quiet slipping away of many a patient whose symptoms are being relieved and who is surrounded by a loving family.

Patients who have learned to trust the doctor may well be able to share these fears and be reassured. But words like "cancer" and "death" are tainted with so many horrific accretions that it may be hard for the patient to use them. We may need to show by our own matter of fact manner that we are not afraid to speak the unspeakable. This does not mean that we should force people to face facts that they are not yet ready to face, but there are many ways in which we can ease things along. By inviting questions, answering honestly the questions that are asked (but not, necessarily, the ones that are not asked), and giving reassurance when reassurance is possible and emotional support to grieving when it is not, we shall often help patients and their families to make something good of the time that remains to them.

Fear often aggravates itself. Thus a person with cancer may lie in bed worrying about his or her cancer. We do not need to read Melzack and Wall's "gate" theory[2] to know that *the gate to pain is opened by fear*; any minor ache or pain will get worse if we worry about it. Many of the pains of cancer patients are not directly caused by cancer but we need to take them seriously, discover their cause, and give an explanation and reassurance that will convince the patient, as well as prescribing appropriate medication, if we are to relieve them.

The list of physical symptoms that can be caused by fear is a long one and ranges from the physiological effects of disturbance of the autonomic nervous system to the secondary effects of overbreathing. When they occur in people who are already physically ill the resulting mixture of physical and psychosomatic symptoms is not always easy to unravel.

Although we often know that a particular case of cancer is likely to end fatally, we can seldom predict how long it will take.[3] One of the hardest problems for us and our patients is *living with uncertainty,* and patients will often demand to be told how long they have to live. *We should not make predictions that will probably be wrong,* and we need to be prepared to support our patients while they wait for the situation to clarify itself.

It is often wise to resist pressure to carry out another operation or another battery of tests the results of which are unlikely to leave the patient any better off. Clearly, if we are to be of help we must tread a line between alarmist overinvestigation and facile reassurance. It is important to diagnose what we can treat, but we need to *know when to stop investigating* and treating the untreatable.

But uncertainty does not mean no treatment. *There is always something that can be done to help* people through the long periods of waiting, be it a regular chat with a trusted general practitioner or oncologist with whom they can air their fears or the prescription of a minor tranquilliser which may break the vicious circle of fear and symptoms. Despite the problems of habituation that limit the value of diazepam it still has a place in the short term treatment of anxiety, particularly in those whose life is not likely to be long enough for habituation to become a problem. Several antidepressants have anxiolytic properties which may benefit

101

people who are anxious and depressed. These include selective serotonin reuptake inhibitors (such as fluoxetine) as well as the more sedative of the tricyclic antidepressant drugs (such as amitriptyline and dothiepin). Finally we should not underestimate the value of the numerous aids to relaxation that are now available.

Cancer invades families, and it is important to reach out to all of those whose lives are touched by it. Thus the *unit of care is the family (which includes the patient)*. Support given to a patient's spouse indirectly helps the patient and may break the vicious circles that arise when fear escalates within a family. That said it is common to find that *as long as the patient is alive the family will minimise their needs* for help and support. We should be aware that things are not always as satisfactory as they seem. A good way to tap into the needs of the family is to invite them to help us to draw *a family tree*. This not only tells us who exists it also demonstrates our interest and allows family members to share their fears and other feelings about each other.

The dying patient's griefs

Although the course of cancers and other fatal diseases can seldom be predicted, they do tend to progress in a stepwise way.

Box 10.2   Losses of patients with life threatening illness

- Loss of security
- Loss of physical functions
- Loss of body image
- Loss of power/strength
- Loss of independence
- Loss of self esteem
- Loss of the respect of others
- Loss of future

Initially the prognosis may not be bad; an operation and a course of radiotherapy or chemotherapy may offer the hope of cure and most patients and doctors prefer to adopt an optimistic attitude. This does not mean that nothing has been lost. Quite apart from the physical mutilation and loss of function that can result from drastic treatments for drastic diseases, patients who have suffered a life threatening illness will never be as secure again as once they were. We need to be at hand and to encourage them to share their perception of the implications of the illness for their life.

The griefs which result from the bodily losses caused by cancer and the surgical procedures to which it gives rise were discussed in chapter 5. *If people have been helped to express their grief at the losses that have occurred at an early stage of an illness they will be more likely to be able to cope effectively when they are faced with another set of losses.* After a period of relative quiescence a new symptom may arise, it is investigated and is found to indicate that the cancer has spread. This time it is more difficult to deny the fact that things are not going the way they should. Perhaps another course of chemotherapy is given but the benefits are less and the patient's general condition is likely to be deteriorating. It becomes obvious that this person will never be able to return to work, and this may be a real cause for grief.

One of the most disturbing losses is the loss of the respect of others, which is reflected in their expressions of pity, for *pity, unlike sympathy, demeans the person pitied.* To some extent this is counteracted if we and the patient's family continue to treat the patient with respect. Conversely it will be aggravated if we patronise, infantilise, or denigrate the patient. Illness may be burdensome to us as well as to our patients. It is important to see the illness as the burden not the patient. Again the provision of emotional support as each of these losses is recognised will increase the chance that the patient will cope successfully with the final stage of the illness when the prospect of death becomes immediate.

The "*stages of dying*" described by Elizabeth Kubler Ross in *Denial, Anger, Bargaining, Depression and Acceptance*[4] bear some resemblance to the phases of grief which were described on pp 19–20; but the griefs of the cancer patient are many and, as Schultz and Aderman have pointed out,[5] the unpredictable way in which most cancers progress means that few follow the neat course outlined by Ross. Even so there is a tendency for people to move in fits and starts from a state of relative denial of the true situation to some kind of acceptance. Some never accept the situation and continue to expect to get better, others seem to embrace the prospect of death. In between there is a majority who oscillate between courageous attempts to face facts and episodes of optimism that are quite unrealistic. The situation is further complicated by people's need to meet the expectations

103

of others; we all want to be seen as a "good patient". This may cause us to conceal some thoughts and feelings and to pretend to others. These fluctuations and obfuscations make it difficult to get reliable measures of "insight" and most research in this field is of dubious value.

Anger and depression, which are common accompaniments of grief, and "bargaining", by which Ross means the attempts which cancer patients often make to accept one sacrifice in the expectation of a reward ("I don't mind losing my hair as long as I can be kept alive until my daughter's wedding"), are often found, although they seldom occur in a particular order.

In the later stages *the loss of all of the appetites*, including the appetite for life, *makes acceptance easier*, and many patients find it easier to "let go" of life because of this.

In all cases the patient's personality and their accustomed ways of viewing the world and coping with problems will colour the way they cope with the problems of illness and death. Those whose experience of life has left them confident in their own worth and trusting in the love of others usually seem to maintain their sense of security in the face of death; others, who may be less secure in both their confidence in themselves and their trust in others (and ultimately in God) may find it hard to step into the unknown. *Spiritual values* which arise from having found meaning in life make it easier to find meaning in death, but this should not be confused with religiosity which is often an attempt to propitiate God and seek his protection. This kind of faith often breaks down when God fails to keep his side of the supposed bargain.

Whatever our own faith may be it is important to respect the faiths of others and to resist the temptation to proselytise. Each person has his or her own religious language, and we must learn that language if we are to communicate successfully on spiritual issues. That said there are many who will enjoy the opportunity to share with us their attempts to make sense of their lives and it is our privilege to be a part of this search.

The doctor's grief

To help those who are dying we must be prepared to get close to them, to share their griefs, and to stay with them in their fear. Sometimes we shall have the satisfaction of knowing that the pain we have shared has been followed by a peaceful and even a triumphant end and this makes it easier to bear, but there are no guarantees. *Sometimes death is a messy and a bitter business which leaves us harrowed and ashamed.* Maybe the person who died has triggered off our own most dreaded fears, maybe we feel responsible for their suffering or their death.

At such times we too will need the support of someone we can trust—and we should not feel ashamed to ask for it. We too will need to grieve, and *if it is all right for our patients to cry it should be all right for us too.* We are not superhumans who can always be counted on to give help but never need it for ourselves, and we must be prepared to let others take over, for a while, the daily routines to give us space to grieve. It is a sign of maturity to know when to ask for help, and the wise doctor will have worked out systems of support to meet a range of needs. This topic is examined in more detail in chapter 13.

The medical team

The mutual support of a team, be it a primary care team, a ward team, or a palliative care team, is never more important than it is for patients, families, and professionals who are facing death. The specialty of palliative medicine has developed so well in recent years that we no longer need to assume that there is nothing that can be done to relieve suffering, physical or mental. Palliative care teams are always happy to give advice, even when they are not directly involved, and there are several other sources of advice available to doctors and patients which are listed in the appendix.

Good control of symptoms is usually the first priority, and it may not be possible to deal with psychological issues until this has been achieved. At the same time the successful relief of pain or other symptoms does more to earn respect and foster trust than anything else. Having proved our worth in one field we shall often find that the patient and family are now more ready to share their thoughts and fears about the other problems they face. It then becomes possible for us to alleviate fear and give reassurance when this is possible and to support people through their grief when it is not.

105

Recommended reading

For a more detailed account of the psychosocial care of the dying a book by a hospice psychiatrist, Averill Stedeford's *Facing Death: Patients, Families and Professionals*, is recommended.[6] For a more comprehensive text book covering the current state of palliative medicine see Doyle, Hanks, and MacDonald.[7]

1 Parkes CM. Attachment and autonomy at the end of life. In: Gosling R, ed. *Support, innovation, and autonomy.* London: Tavistock, 1973:151–66.
2 Melzack R, Wall PD. Pain mechanisms. *Science* 1965;150:971–9.
3 Parkes CM. Accuracy of predictions of survival in later stages of cancer. *BMJ* 1972;ii:29–31.
4 Ross EK. *On death and dying.* London: Tavistock, 1970.
5 Schulz R, Aderman D. Clinical research and the stages of dying. *Omega* 1974; 5:137–43.
6 Stedeford A. *Facing death: patients, families and professionals.* London: Heinemann, 1984.
7 Doyle D, Hanks GWC, MacDonald N, eds. *Oxford textbook of palliative medicine.* 2nd ed. Oxford: Oxford University Press, 1998.

11 The dying child and bereaved parent

DORA BLACK

The terminal phase of a life threatening illness may be defined as one when curative treatments are not applicable but palliation is given. There is evidence that *children, even young ones, are usually aware that they are dying.* They may pick up these cues from parents and from hospital staff, who in one study gave significantly less time and attention to children who were terminally ill than to others.[1] They may not let anyone know that they know. Child and parents may maintain a "mutual pretence"[2] and yet families who have open communication fare better psychologically. *The refusal of parents and medical carers to talk about issues of death and dying with children who have life threatening diseases impedes coping for the whole family.*[3]

Parents appreciate staff openness and many years later remember the method of imparting the bad news vividly. Accurate information delivered with skill and sympathy and updated regularly lessens the parents' sense of helplessness and isolation and sets up a therapeutic alliance.[4]

Treatment setting

Children can be treated in a hospital ward, in a hospice for children, or at home. Parents are more anxious, depressed, and defensive after death in hospital than at home, and *when children die at home* the long term outcome is better for the parents,[5] although the reactions of siblings have not been similarly studied.

Although *children's hospices* have been in existence for only a short time, they do have a specific role and can be helpful in providing respite care. When death at home is not an option

107

because of the complex medical and nursing needs of the child or because of factors such as the needs of siblings or others they can provide terminal care.[6] More specialist units are developing home care teams so that children can receive much of their terminal care at home. Results of preliminary studies are encouraging.[7,8]

Effects on siblings

Siblings' understanding of illness seems to be related to age. Delays in understanding concepts compared with understanding in families with healthy children, may be caused by avoidance of discussion of illness in families with sick children.[9]

Siblings of dying children have about double the risk of developing psychological disturbance; this seems to be related to demographic characteristics of the family, level of family functioning, and characteristics of the disease. Knowledge of illness is different in siblings of ill children compared with siblings of healthy children. Nevertheless, most siblings of sick children seem to be well adjusted and do not have psychiatric disorders. Most of the studies, however, have been cross sectional and have not looked at long term effects. Clinical experience suggests that preventive intervention counselling should be offered to all siblings of dying children.

Effects on parents

Mothers, more than fathers, are involved in nursing and caring for dying children and have therefore been more extensively studied. In several studies mothers have been found to suffer in excess from depression.[10,11] Mothers have reported a greater degree of difficulty with the problems of helplessness, loss of confidence in the ability to be a good parent, financial difficulties, being avoided by others, growing apart from their spouse, and fear of being unable to cope if the child should die than have fathers, who reported significantly greater difficulty with two problems—feeling left out of the ill child's life and later being worried that their spouse was too preoccupied with the dead child.[12]

In a systematic 8 year follow up study Lundin found more evidence of persisting tearfulness and grieving among parents who had lost a child than among widows and widowers,[13] but the widows and widowers were more likely to continue to think about their dead partner and to express feelings of guilt. Parents may feel that they can never recover fully from the loss of a child; they may adjust to it, they may be able to resume their everyday activities and may even derive pleasure from life, but they feel they remain vulnerable.[14] For some parents the new identity is a stronger one—they feel they have been "through the fire" and that nothing can affect them so profoundly again. The cost may be a reduction in their sensitivity to their other children or their partner, which may threaten the marriage or even disrupt it.

Effects on marriage

Marriages and similar relationships are stressed by the demands of treatment for serious illness and by the death of a child. Often the treating specialist hospital is at a distance, and parents are separated as one accompanies the child and the other tries to keep the rest of the family going and earn a living. It is surprising therefore that most studies have not found an increase in divorce or separation, although marital distress is increased and this becomes worse as the disease worsens.[15] *It seems that the stress of a serious and prolonged illness in a child is likely to make a poor marriage worse but may strengthen the relationship in an already close marriage, thus balancing the statistics.*

A study of long term adjustment in families of children with cancer compared 38 families of a child who survived 5 years after treatment had ended with 13 families whose child had died. Five years after the death, the families of children who died scored at less adaptive levels of functioning on items that measured return to normal activities, zest for living, making plans for the future, recognising and accepting the family members' needs, admitting the need for emotional support from friends or family, and having placed the cancer in a more reasonable and less overwhelming perspective.[16]

Another study looked at the coping strategies of parents of children with cancer and found that they were not related to income or sex.[17] Parents who had a good relationship with the medical staff tended to use coping strategies such as denial, acceptance, or reliance on religion. More highly educated parents tended to use information seeking as a coping strategy.

Death of a fetus or neonate

Miscarriages, induced termination of pregnancy, and stillbirths all provoke a grief reaction. It is likely that the degree of grief is directly related to the length of gestation and to whether it was a wanted child.[18] Ultrasound imaging of the fetus has resulted in earlier recognition of its humanity and may have increased the likelihood of a more severe grief reaction. *Viewing the stillborn baby aids the resolution of grief,* as does a proper burial or cremation ceremony. Most women who spontaneously miscarry or have a stillbirth or neonatal death feel inadequate and a failure in their reproductive function and would benefit from counselling.

Many deaths in the first 4 weeks of life are related to congenital abnormalities in the infant, and parents need much support and informed advice, including genetic counselling, before they embark on further pregnancies.[19,20] The sudden infant death syndrome (SIDS) is the commonest cause of infant death between 4 and 52 weeks of age and causes high distress because of its suddenness, unexpectedness, and unknown aetiology.[21]

Helping the family of a dying child

The primary health care team may feel side lined when a child has a terminal illness. These deaths are so rare, and the treatment of the life threatening illness which may have preceded the terminal phase may have been in the hands of specialists in a distant hospital who may have maintained only formal and minimal contact with the general practitioner. One study found that *family doctors rarely inquire about family functioning when a child is ill.*[22] Caring for a dying child at home will inevitably involve family doctors more, and parents appreciate the interest expressed by their practitioner even if he or she cannot cure their child.

The health visitor or practice nurse or the general practitioners themselves might find the time to pay a regular visit to the family or invite them to the surgery to review the functioning of each member of the family, attend to communication within the family, especially with the children, and check that all the social benefits to which the family are entitled are being claimed. As death draws near there needs to be an increase in the emotional care of the family, ensuring that the children have been informed of what is likely to happen, and that there is a mobilisation of family and

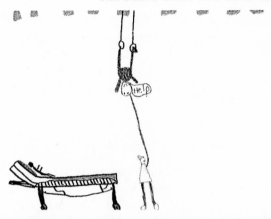

Figure 11.1   This was drawn by a 10 year old boy with a brain tumour. He described it as depicting him lying in bed and seeing himself suspended from the ceiling with the nurse manipulating him with the noose tied in a rope. His therapist worked with him on his feelings of helplessness engendered by his illness and the treatments for it. Note the accurate perception of the hospital bed.

neighbourhood support. A review of the effects of bereavement on the different members of the family is helpful in calming the bereaved person's fears that his or her experiences foreshadow insanity. Siblings will usually benefit from being included in the viewing rituals and the funeral but need proper preparation and explanation beforehand. They need to understand the permanence of death.

Counsellors must respect the religious beliefs of the family and be prepared to discuss with parents how they can communicate with their surviving children. For example, in Christian families, it is important that children understand that it is not the dead body that goes to heaven but that the parents believe that the dead child's soul is in heaven. Souls can exist only in a live person. When the body of that person dies, the soul flies off to heaven to live with God. Since the child's soul hasn't got a body to live in, he or she cannot return to earth.

When a death during pregnancy occurs, parents in their distress may omit to let the siblings know what has happened. The children may have been told that mummy is having a baby and then no baby appears. The family practitioner could *check that the children know what has happened and why and that it was not their fault.*

One controlled study has shown that *brief counselling can significantly reduce morbidity* in parents after a perinatal death.[23] A

111

useful source of advice is to be found in a paper by White and colleagues.[24] The Stillbirth and Neonatal Death Society (SANDS), the Compassionate Friends, and the Foundation for the Study of Infant Death offer volunteer counselling in many parts of Britain as does Cruse Bereavement Care. For further details of these organisations see the appendix.

Continuing education for the primary care team

Do general practitioners and their teams need more training in understanding the psychosocial aspects of children and death and the techniques of bereavement counselling? While many general practitioners are comfortable in talking to adults about their impending death, they may feel less comfortable in talking with children. Some medical schools are tackling this problem with courses on communicating with children and on bereavement counselling, and many general practitioner training courses have at least one lecture on the subject.[25-29] Cruse Bereavement Care and other organisations run courses on bereavement counselling.

Recommended reading

Goldman's *Care of the Dying Child* is an excellent small book which deals comprehensively with the physical, psychological, and spiritual management of different terminal illnesses in children, paying attention to the care of the family and the professional carers.[30]

1 Waechter EH. Children's awareness of fatal illness. *Am J Nursing* 1971;7: 1168–72.
2 Bluebond-Langner M. *The private worlds of dying children*. Princeton, New Jersey: Princeton University Press, 1978.
3 Slavin L, O'Malley J, Koocher G, *et al.* Communication of the cancer diagnosis to pediatric patients: impact on long-term adjustment. *Am J Psychiatry* 1982; **139**:179–83.
4 Woolley H, Stein A, Forrest G, *et al.* Imparting the diagnosis of life threatening illness in children. *BMJ* 1989;**298**:1623–6.
5 Lauer ME, Mulhern RK, Schell MJ, *et al.* Long-term follow-up of parental adjustment following a child's death at home or hospital. *Cancer* 1989;**63**: 988–94.

6 Stein A, Woolley H. An evaluation of hospice care for children. In: Baum JD, Dominica F, Woodward RN, eds. *Listen, my child has a lot of living to do.* Oxford: Oxford University Press, 1990.

7 Martinson IM. Home care for the dying child with cancer: feasibility and desirability. *Loss, Grief and Care* 1986;**1**:97–114

8 Chambers EJ, Oakhill A, Cornish JM, *et al.* Terminal care at home for children with cancer. *BMJ* 1989;**298**:937–40.

9 Caradang MLA, Folkins CH, Hines PA, *et al.* The role of cognitive level and sibling illness in children's conceptualizations of illness. *Am J Orthopsychiat* 1979;**49**:474–81.

10 Daniels D, Miller JJ, Billings AG, *et al.* Psychosocial risk and resistance factors among children with chronic illness, healthy siblings, and healthy controls. *J Abnormal Child Psychol* 1987;**15**:295–308.

11 Jessop DJ, Riessman CK, Stein REK. Chronic childhood illness and maternal mental health. *J Dev Behav Pediatrics* 1988;**9**:147–56.

12 Cooke JA. Influence of gender on the problems of parents of fatally ill children. *J Psychosoc Oncol* 1984;**2**:71–91.

13 Lundin T. Long term outcome of bereavement. *Br J Psychiatry* 1984;**145**:424–8.

14 Osterweis M, Solomon F, Green M. *Bereavement: reactions, consequences and care.* Washington, DC: National Academy Press, 1984.

15 Sabbeth B, Leventhal J. Marital adjustment to chronic childhood illness: a critique of the literature. *Pediatrics* 1984;**73**:762–7.

16 Spinetta JJ, Murphy JL, Vik PJ, *et al.* Long-term adjustment in families of children with cancer. Special Issue: clinical research issues in psychosocial oncology. *J Psychosoc Oncol* 1988;**6**:179–91.

17 Barbarin OA, Chesler M. The medical context of parental coping with childhood cancer. *Am J Community Psychol* 1986;**14**:221–35.

18 Davidson GW. Stillbirth, neonatal death and sudden infant death syndrome. In: Wass H, Corr CA, eds. *Childhood and death.* Washington, DC: Hemisphere, 1995:243–60.

19 Stewart M. Programs for intervention after a perinatal death. *Birth Defects* 1987;**23**:52–5.

20 Theut SK, Zaslow MJ, Rabinovich BA, *et al.* Resolution of parental bereavement after a perinatal loss. *J Am Acad Child Adolsec Psychiatry* 1990;**29**:521–5.

21 Ostfeld BM, Ryan T, Hiatt M, *et al.* Maternal grief after sudden infant death syndrome. *J Develop Behav Pediat* 1993;**14**:156–62.

22 Rosser JE, Maguire P. Dilemmas in general practice; the care of the cancer patient. *Soc Sci Med* 1982;**16**:315–22.

23 Forrest GC, Standish E, Baum JD. Support after perinatal death: a study of support and counselling after perinatal bereavement. *BMJ* 1982;**285**:1475–9.

24 White MP, Reynolds B, Evans TJ. Handling of death in special care nurseries and parental grief. *BMJ* 1984;**289**:167–9.

25 Black D, Hardoff D, Nelki J. Educating medical students about death and dying. *Arch Dis Child* 1989;**64**:750–3.

26 Bleeker JAC, Pomerantz HB. The influence of a lecture course in loss and grief on medical students: an empirical study of attitude formation. *Medical Education* 1979;**13**:117–28.

27 Bloch S. Instruction on death and dying for medical student. *Medical Education* 1976;**10**:269–73.

28 Field D. Formal instruction in UK medical schools about death and dying. *Medical Education* 1984;**18**:429–34.

29 Howells K, Gould M, Field D. Fear of death and dying in medical students: effects of clinical experience. *Medical Education* 1986;**20**:502–6.

30 Goldman A, ed. *Care of the dying child.* Oxford: Oxford University Press, 1994.

12 Disasters

COLIN MURRAY PARKES AND DORA BLACK

Although most people in the West now live in a world which is safer than it has ever been, the very scale of our technological society and the density of the populations in which we live mean that when things do go wrong the consequences can be literally disastrous. A Boeing 747 crashes on a town, a ferry overturns, a football stadium catches fire, a rush hour train crashes—any of these happenings can bring about a high mortality in a short space of time and all of them have happened in the United Kingdom in recent years.

These disasters and others like them have provided us with opportunities to learn a great deal about the psychological consequences of small and medium scale disasters and have led to much research and the proposal of several plans for mitigating the effects of future disasters. In Britain they have given rise to the inception of a Civil Emergencies Secretariat at the Home Office and a government sponsored working party who produced a report and an action plan.[1]

In other countries natural disasters are still common, and these sometimes occur on a very large scale. Earthquakes, tornadoes, and floods affecting large cities can kill huge numbers of people and overwhelm any local emergency services and sources of psychosocial support. At the other extreme we have the numerous small scale disasters that result from terrorist attacks, motorway pile ups, and the collapse of buildings or bridges. These merge with the other causes of violent death which exist in every society.

Clearly *no one plan is likely to be suitable for all disasters*, and books such as those by Raphael[2] and Hodgkinson and Stewart[3] cover a range of scenarios. It will not be possible here to do more than give an outline of this large topic and to point out some of the general implications. All other chapters in this book are relevant to disaster work because of the wide range of losses that can result.

114

Psychological consequences of disasters

Disasters often give rise to the very conditions that place traumatised and bereaved people at special psychological risk. They include the

---

Box 12.1   Factors contributing to psychological risk after disasters

- Witnessing or experiencing horrific or terrifying events or injuries
- Major threat to life
- Suffering unexpected losses
- Suffering multiple losses
- Prior psychological vulnerability

---

effects of witnessing or experiencing terrifying events, suffering serious injuries, and, suddenly and unexpectedly, losing people and possessions to whom we are attached. Terrifying or horrific events tend to give rise to haunting memories which may amount to a post-traumatic stress disorder (PTSD), unexpected losses give rise to grief which may become pathological, and physical injuries can cause both grief for the lost part and its functions and anxiety states. Some unfortunate people may suffer all of these consequences. Furthermore, because disasters affect large numbers of people there are bound to be some among them who were vulnerable to stress before the disaster struck. It should not surprise us to find that *there is a need for counselling and psychiatric services in the aftermath.*

The sequence from impact to recoil to a post-traumatic period is a useful way of viewing the consequences and planning services.[4]

Impact

Disasters differ from other types of trauma in their scale and their effects on the *sources of support* to whom we normally turn at times of stress and loss. Thus families may be wiped out or so stricken that, for a while, their members are unable to support each other; members of the care giving professions may themselves be traumatised or bereaved, and homes, hospitals, and health centres may be destroyed. At the same time disasters often attract a flood of well meaning outsiders who may obstruct the attempts of the professionals to act effectively. Chaos reigns and it is difficult for anyone, in the short term, to get a focus on what is needed. This is reflected in the "illusion of centrality", which causes people on the periphery of a disaster area to imagine that they are in the centre and to demand an unfair share of the caring resources.

An *immediate reaction of numbness* is to be expected along with high levels of anxiety and an urgent need to "do something" even when there is nothing to be done. Attempts at rescue are often continued long after it is clear that there is no hope of success, and people may exhaust themselves to the point that they do more harm than good and need to be gently removed from the scene. This said, one should not underestimate the heroism and self sacrifice that takes place and may help to overcome enormous difficulties. Nobody who works in a disaster area can fail to be impressed by the good will and unsolicited help that pours in. The problem is to get it organised.

Bewilderment is a prominent reaction and some of those most affected by the trauma may suffer amnesia, fugue states, or other dissociative phenomena. Panic is rare but may take place if people believe themselves to be trapped.

Recoil

Once the emergency is at an end and the rescue services have withdrawn, painful feelings, which have been repressed up to now, begin to emerge. Intense grief, anger, and guilt at having survived are to be expected along with high levels of persisting anxiety as if *everyone were waiting for the next disaster* to take place. Some plummet into depression and may even be at risk of suicide. There is a great pressure to talk about what has happened, and survivors feel a need to relate their experiences again and again.

This is the time when *plans need to be made*, but this may be hard when feelings are running high and anger is often being misdirected at anyone who tries to take a lead. There is a strongly felt need to find culprits who can be blamed for the disaster, rumours are rife, and public meetings easily degenerate into brawls. Scapegoating is common and can be very unfair. Would be helpers who have burnt their fingers may then withdraw and necessary decisions be postponed. *A paralysis of decision making* may result.

On the positive side disasters often generate *a sense of cohesion* and caring within a community that may draw together people who would not normally commit themselves to community action.

116

The good will generated by the disaster may bring in resources of people and money from outside the community that enable plans to be carried out. This, in its turn, may evoke the jealousy of others who lack such resources.

Post-traumatic period

Because the reactions to a disaster are so various it is not possible to make accurate predictions of the time a community will take to recover. *Factors which can contribute to recovery or failure to recover* in a community include the existence of support systems from inside and outside the community, the judicial processes which follow every disaster and are of particular importance when it was caused by people, the rituals of memorialisation, and the image of itself that the community obtains via the mass media.

The judicial process is often painfully slow and can delay recovery, but it is always important that justice is seen to be done and every effort needs to be made to convince those affected by the disaster that their views will be heard and that no "whitewash" will take place. Compensation and the disaster funds which are set up after disasters allow the populace to express their sympathy and carry a symbolic significance that transcends their monetary value. What seems to be indecorous bickering between traumatised people may, in fact, reflect the deep feelings evoked by moneys that are seen as rewards or tributes to the dead.

Even in a secular society the *rituals* occasioned by disasters carry deep significance. These range from official visits by important people to memorial services and more permanent memorials to the dead. They reduce the general feeling of helplessness and provide the traumatised and the bereaved with social support, sanction for grief, and opportunities to find meaning in their lives and in the lives of those who have died. They also help people to find new places for the dead. This does not represent a denial of loss but a recognition and way of symbolising the truth of the words "He (or she) lives on in my memory".

Those who have witnessed horrific events or been terrified by threats to their own lives are particularly vulnerable to the *persistence of painful memories* along with high levels of anxiety and hypervigilance (with a tendency to startle easily). This may be so severe that it causes sufferers to avoid any situation or person who will remind them of the trauma. They may give up work, shut

117

themselves up at home, and refuse to talk about what has happened.

These are symptoms of *post-traumatic stress disorder*[5] and it can be very disabling. The formal psychiatric definition is given in

---

Box 12.2 Diagnostic features of post-traumatic stress disorder (after diagnostic statistical manual, IV)

A Experience of being confronted with actual or threatened death or serious injury of self or others and reaction of intense fear, helplessness, or horror

B Traumatic event persistently re-experienced as intrusive memories, repeated distressing dreams, flashbacks (reliving the experience), intense distress at reminders, and/or physiological reactivity to cues reflecting the traumatic event

C Persistent avoidance of reminders or numbing including at least three of the following: efforts to avoid thoughts or feelings associated with the trauma; efforts to avoid people, places, or activities associated with the trauma; amnesia for aspects of the trauma; loss of interest or participation in activities; feelings of detachment or estrangement from others; inability to feel; loss of faith in the future

D Persistent symptoms of increased arousal including at least two of the following: insomnia; irritability; poor concentration; hypervigilance; and/or exaggerated startle response

E Disturbance persists for more than a month

F Disturbance causes clinically significant distress or impairment of functioning

---

box 12.2. Despite their efforts to avoid reminders, the memories repeatedly return to haunt people, both during their waking hours and often also at night in the form of nightmares. To avoid thinking about something we have to think about it, to hold it in mind at some level. The sufferer is therefore unable to let go of the painful facts of loss and unable to find a way to live with them.

Children who witness sudden horrific deaths are particularly likely to suffer post-traumatic stress disorder. As in adults disturbing images and memories of the event are imprinted and return unbidden. The event may be re-experienced in full as a *"flash back"* in response to environmental triggers or memories.

If their most recent and imprinted image of a loved person acts as a traumatic reminder, both children and adults may try to put this out of their mind and consequently the grieving process is impeded.[6] Recurrent nightmares in which the traumatic events are replayed without alteration are particularly common and begin to include elements of the person's wishes and fantasies only as the person finds ways of coping with the trauma and can begin to grieve.

The nightmares of trauma are always distressing and may prevent say, a child who has witnessed the murder of a parent, dreaming more calmly about the dead parent and gaining comfort from the feeling that he or she is near. These dreams, "grief dreams", seem to help in coming to terms with the loss. Intrusive daytime recollections also interfere with the child's efforts to remember the dead parent. The mutilated image prevents reminiscence in tranquillity. Traumatic play can be repetitive and uncreative and interfere with the use of play to confront and work through grief. In the fortunately rare but extreme cases where a child witnesses the death of a parent or sibling at the hands of the other parent and the children suffer in addition to their loss(es) dislocation, conflicted loyalties, and continuing anxiety the outcome is often grave.[7]

Clinical experience indicates that symptoms of post-traumatic stress disorder can be prevented or mitigated by a swift intervention that helps the person to understand the traumatic events and moves him or her into mourning.

Box 12.3   Disaster care

- Preparation and planning
- Impact and emergency care
- Recoil—debriefing, appraisal, mobilisation of resources, training disaster team
- Post-traumatic period—outreach, counselling, treatment

Preparing for disasters

Although many of the disasters that have taken place in recent years have led to effective *programmes of support, these have always taken too long to organise* and sufficient help has seldom been given when it was most needed—during the first few weeks after the disaster. These delays can be minimised if plans are made in advance.

Most of the skills that are needed to help people affected by disasters are no different from the *skills that are needed after other traumatic life events. They should be part of the basic training of every doctor* and many other members of the caring professions. Sadly there are few courses of basic training that give proper attention to these issues and most professionals will benefit from post-basic training in trauma and bereavement counselling.

In Britain the people with local responsibility for psychosocial care in disasters are the directors of social services. The Working Party on Disasters recommends that these directors should liaise with medical and other services in their areas before disasters occur to make plans and reduce delays.[1] People with training in trauma and bereavement counselling *should be included* in all disaster plans and should be given the opportunity to practise these skills in disaster exercises.

Responding to disasters

Impact

After the impact of a disaster the immediate need is to save lives, and this must take priority over psychosocial care. Local organisations such as the Womens' Royal Voluntary Service (WRVS) can usually be counted on to provide the tea and emotional support that is needed, leaving members of the medical profession free to assist in the rescue operation.

It is important for us to remember that *rescue workers may exhaust themselves and "burn out"*. We may be the only ones with sufficient authority to insist that carers who have come to the end of their tether take a rest, and we must be prepared to give emergency psychiatric care when it is needed.

Benzodiazepines such as diazepam still have a place in the treatment of acute traumatic stress reactions, panic syndrome, and dissociative syndromes. They can be given by injection if necessary. It is wise to limit the prescription to one or a few doses because of the dangers of habituation.

120

Recoil

This is the time to firm up and implement plans, and the first step must be an *accurate appraisal of the situation* with a view to establishing who is in need of psychosocial support and how this can be provided (for a more detailed account of the planning process see Parkes[8]). This will be determined by the *scale* and *spread* of the disaster, two characteristics that do not necessarily go together. Thus disasters may be of small (say 10–100 deaths), medium (100–1000 deaths), or large scale (1000 and more deaths) and may affect victims from a narrow (local) or wide (regional, national, or international) spread. A small local disaster can often be managed by existing services with no more than advisory help from outside the district. Even medium scale disasters may be managed by local services if the victims' homes are spread over a wide area. On the other hand medium scale local disasters are bound to overstretch existing local services and help will need to be mobilised from outside the locality. Large scale disasters are likely to require help across international boundaries. Regardless of scale, disasters with spread over a wide geographical area create special problems in the coordination of help across boundaries, and this makes it more difficult to set up a coordinated disaster plan.

Box 12.4   Categories of people for whom help may need to be organised

- Casualties—injured Survivors
- Uninjured survivors
- Bereaved relatives and friends
- Bystanders
- Members of rescue and other support services
- Secondary victims (for example, people who believe themselves to be at risk of similar disasters)

Some people will fall into more than one of these categories

Indispensable to any disaster response is the early setting up of *a computerised database* to record the names and other particulars of the dead, of all persons recognised as being at potential risk, and of all those who offer help. An office with sufficient telephone lines and operators to deal with the flood of calls that are bound to come in must be set up and the phone number advertised widely through the media.

Having identified the categories of people at risk and made a preliminary estimate of the number who will need help it is then necessary to assess the number and types of helper needed. Local social service departments can be expected to take a lead, but it is extremely unlikely that their busy staff will be able to take on more than a small part of the case load produced by a disaster and they must work in cooperation with other statutory and voluntary agencies.

In most localities general practitioners and other members of the primary care team will have important parts to play. Many of those who are suffering post-traumatic stress disorder or other psychological symptoms will seek their help, often with somatic complaints. Close liaison with the disaster team is necessary if duplication of service is to be avoided, and this can usually be carried out with permission and without breaching the patient's rights to confidentiality. Health centres and surgeries are useful sources of information to those at risk. Information about the disaster plan and the support services available should be circulated and displayed.

An important action during the recoil stage is the *debriefing* of members of the emergency services who are now being stood down. This has the dual purpose of providing emotional support to people who may have suffered frustration, danger, and the witnessing of horrific events and providing them with the opportunity to report back and to take part in the planning process. Doctors and others in positions of leadership carry daunting responsibilities at such times and are likely to need support. Unfortunately they are also the least likely to ask for it. All disaster plans should cover this problem.

A Press Officer should be appointed to liaise with the media, who are a valuable source of help if used wisely but also capable of intrusive exploitation of traumatised and bereaved people.

Post-traumatic period

Because of the special risks to the mental health of many of those affected by disasters it is necessary to be *proactive in offering help to all who are deemed to be at risk*. Rather than waiting for people at risk to "break down" we need to reach out to them and make sure that they are fully informed of the help that is available to them. In most disaster plans *a team of trained counsellors* will be mobilised from such organisations as Cruse Bereavement Care, Relate, Victim Support Schemes, etc. (see appendix). They are the front line of supporters who need to be backed up by psychologists, psychiatrists, social workers, psychotherapists, and others with special training and skills. Doctors will often be a person's first choice of helper, and they need to decide whether or not, in particular cases, they have the skills and the time that is needed to provide the counselling. This said one cannot underestimate the value of one or two interviews with a doctor, which not only enable the doctor to assess the need for further help but, in many cases, will provide all the help that is needed. Reassurance of the normality of many of the symptoms of anxiety which worry people under stress, information about the ways in which a loved person may have died, or simply the opportunity to off load feelings of grief, anger, or guilt may be all that a traumatised person needs or wants from us.

A multidisciplinary *day conference* is a useful way to take stock and to provide some extra training by professionals with experience of disaster work to all of those who are providing support to bereaved and traumatised people. This should be in addition to the regular supervision and support required. It is a reflection on the training of doctors that we imagine that, unlike other human beings, we have no need for such support.

A key issue is the *management of traumatic memories*. Here it is important to help people to realise that, while attempts to avoid memories are bound to fail, when we choose to think about a painful topic we gain control of it. This is most obvious in the treatment of recurrent nightmares. The aim is not to prevent the dream but to encourage the sufferer to think of a different and more satisfactory ending. When they do this they take control of the dream and lose their fear of it. When the sufferer stops dreading the dream, the dream often stops recurring. The very act of telling another person about a traumatic experience helps the traumatised person to regain control of the situation.

People who meet the criteria for post-traumatic stress disorder given in box 12.2 should be diagnosed and treated as this disorder can easily become chronic if it is not treated promptly and effectively. Also, although grief *per se* is not grounds for compensation, post-traumatic stress disorder is. It may respond to

123

a serotonin reuptake inhibitor such as fluoxetine or to specialised psychological treatments such as eye movement desensitisation. In all cases careful records should be kept as post-traumatic stress disorder and other psychiatric consequences of disasters often lead to claims for compensation for any costs incurred in diagnosis and treatment.

Although most of those affected by disasters will not suffer lasting psychiatric ill health, the need for counselling is likely to continue for at least a year and probably longer. Needs vary and the teams that have been set up should be phased out gradually as the needs diminish rather than being abruptly terminated. When a community has been affected by a disaster it is likely that an enterprise that started as therapeutic will end as something different. Both the members of the disaster team and the traumatised communities they serve are likely to be *profoundly and permanently changed* by the experience of a disaster. They emerge tougher, older, and, sometimes, wiser than they were. Perhaps they will never again feel the comfortable illusion of security that causes most of us to believe that disasters happen only to other people. They are also likely to end up more sensitive to the needs of others and more committed to the deeper meaning of "community".

Further reading

The *Allen Report* was published as an advisory document to assist members of the caring profession to prepare for the psychosocial care of people affected by disasters.[1] It provides a useful set of practical guidelines which have, at this time, been implemented in only a few areas. For a more comprehensive view of the current state of our knowledge of traumatic stress and its consequences, which includes but is not limited to disasters, see Black *et al.*[9]

1 Allen AJ. *Disaster: planning for a caring response*. Part 1 and 2. London: HMSO, 1991.
2 Raphael B. *When disaster strikes*. New York: Basic Books, 1986.
3 Hodgkinson PE, Stewart M. *Coping with catastrophe: a handbook of disaster management*. London: Routledge, 1991.
4 Tyhurst JS. Individual reactions to community disasters: the natural history of psychic phenomena. *Am J Psychiat* 1951;167:764.

5 American Psychiatric Association. *Diagnostic and statistical manual of mental disorders*. 4th ed. (DSM-IV). Washington, DC: American Psychiatric Association, 1994.

6 Pynoos RS, Eth S. Witness to violence: the child interview. *J Am Acad Child Psychiatry* 1986;**25**:306–19.

7 Harris Hendriks J, Black D, Kaplan T. *When father kills mother: guiding children through trauma and grief*. London: Routledge, 1993.

8 Parkes CM. Planning for the aftermath. *J R Soc Med* 1991;**84**:22–5.

9 Black D, Newman M, Harris-Hendriks J, *et al*. eds. *Psychological trauma: A developmental approach*. London: Gaskell, 1997.

13 The doctor's losses: ideals versus realities

GLIN BENNET

After five years of study, newly qualified doctors may find it hard to realise that much of their future development will involve loss. They will go on gathering information and acquiring skills, but if they are to retain their enthusiasm and to mature as people, they will be learning to live with various losses.

Tiredness

New doctors should enjoy the initial enthusiasm, the ideals and the sense of omnipotence and invulnerability, the buoyant feeling of being able to contribute to the general good, because it may not last for long. Very likely a few months of broken nights will blur the ideals and push the ambitions into the distance. The immediate objective becomes to get through the job.

The grinding tiredness teaches them a lot: about their limitations, that sleep matters, and that it is difficult to be a good doctor when their eyes will not stay open. They become impatient over explanations, and tiredness comes up like a barrier so that they can no longer reach out to anxious and grieving patients.

They are learning that they cannot meet the ideals they set for themselves or the expectations of others. But tiredness is cured by a good sleep and enthusiasm is restored by a relaxing weekend. They can be admired for the long hours they work. They work harder than other people, they work amid the basic crises of living, they know about suffering, they see that people get better through their individual efforts, though they are not successful all the time. The death of a patient is a loss that reminds doctors of their limitations and the limitations of medical science, in which they had been taught to have so much faith. The first time it happens,

126

the doctor is sad, shocked, perhaps angry that the patient could have done that to them.

Loss of unreality

Most doctors have relatively simple lives in these early years, so it is possible, if they want, to give all their waking hours to the work in hand. Then there comes a time when the work is not sufficiently sustaining on its own—at least it ceases to be for most people, especially when the needs of others have to be considered. Now the people with the idealism and enthusiasm are confronted with a fresh reality, and *much of a doctor's subsequent life and career will depend on how this matter is addressed.*

This is a further lesson in the loss of omnipotence, but in no way is it the beginning of a decline. It is a time for redirecting the energy. Doctors who accomplish this and can control the circumstances of their work can have a satisfying life, because medicine offers such abundant opportunities.

Many doctors make choices that put them in the front line, where they are directly exposed to needy members of the public. Here, the external pressures may seem always to be about to overwhelm them. The ideals are abandoned, and the redirection cannot be achieved. The giving out exceeds the individual's restorative powers. If as established doctors we find ourselves perpetually rushing to catch up with the demand as we see it, if our families tell us that we are irritable and our friends that we look tired all the time, then we are letting our resources become depleted: the signs of burnout will appear.

There is a phrase: "*You have to be on fire before you can burn out.*" The idealism is gradually replaced by a mild cynicism, patients are perceived as inconsiderate and ungrateful, the telephone becomes an enemy. The process is familiar and, if unchecked, leads on to an apathy, in which minimum energy goes into the clinical work, although it may be redirected into administrative and extracurricular activities.

Men and women have different experiences

The traditional male approach has been to disregard these issues, at the outset of his career or later, and carry on up the professional ladder, regardless of personal considerations. If he becomes powerful enough he can sustain this style of life and put off his maturing, possibly for ever. Sadly, *these are qualities that make for professional success,* and such people can be found among the more influential teachers of medical students, who are thereby exposed to the model of brashness and emotional immaturity.

Women doctors often experience loss before they qualify. They are affected more than most men by the brutalising aspect of medical education, which diminishes the empathic part of clinical work. They delay childbearing to their late 20s or beyond, and then they have to work that much harder to achieve the same professional goals as men.

Loss of meaning, loss of spirit

In the professional man's progress there are critical points, or hurdles, that can be cleared successively and that set him fair for the next stage. The loss of omnipotence is a necessary first stage. Another critical time for men comes in their late 30s, when they usually have their consultant post or their partnership in general practice. They are probably married with children, have a house, a good car, and a boat as well perhaps. The challenge here is that there are no more explicit challenges, such as qualifications and jobs; they have all been attained. Thus, there is a loss of these defining events and the excitement about all that is one day going to be. The doctor wakes one morning and says: "My life is now. This is what I am." This is the plateau of middle life.

High achievers imagine, albeit subconsciously, that the only way on from the plateau is downhill, and that once they have reached a particular professional peak there can only be loss of status, loss of role, diminishing health, and so on down. *The losses are real, but like all losses they are points of transition, which can be seized creatively.* There are gains from this new state: it is no longer necessary to meet all the expectations of others, to keep on achieving or publishing; it is no longer necessary to be wise and in control. There is more time. Life can broaden out at this point, provided that the losses are understood and seen for what they really are.

Women suffer loss in the process of becoming doctors, but there are great benefits later on, and unfulfilled male doctors could learn from their female colleagues. A woman doctor has professional work that she enjoys and often she has a family; thus she is not looking solely to her job to give her a life that is meaningful. Male doctors can do the same, only so often they avoid their families.

Doctors going wrong

When their life can no longer be defined by achievement, doctors often fail to cope. The work has lost its meaning because there is simply too much of it or because the doctor has not adapted to changing circumstances. The issues of omnipotence and invulnerability appear again, but in a more subtle form: it is no longer a matter of one not being able to accomplish everything, but rather accepting that one is merely a vulnerable human being. This comes hard to powerful doctors, and they may try to avoid the transition in various ways: by blotting it out (through alcohol); by reassuring themselves of their potency (by a new relationship); by channelling their energies in new directions (by getting on the train to London, where the important committees meet); by developing symptoms and becoming depressed.

Most problems that doctors experience in middle life are essentially problems of meaning, and their lives have lost their meaning because they have not been able to make the fundamental transitions and to value themselves simply for being who they are.

What is to be done?

It is good that schemes have been organised whereby doctors in difficulties can get confidential help at a distance from their places of work (see appendix), but there is a measure of failure here. Doctors become involved in such schemes because they have not been able to share their deeper feelings with their immediate colleagues, or because problems have been neglected until the situation is out of hand and the doctor is ceasing to function competently.

These doctors are stranded. They have of course lost their omnipotence and invulnerability; and they are no longer climbing the ladder to success, but these losses are denied by them, so they are unable to make the essential transitions. It is as if they can accept themselves only as immaculate and all-competent professionals, and any blemish on that image is seen as a failure.

In fact the blemishes have the potential to be a great advantage, and these doctors would do well to attend to the ancient idea that *only the wounded physician heals.* In myth it is presented in a literal form, but in ordinary life the "wounded" state refers merely to the acceptance of one's imperfections.

When doctors can accept their blemishes and vulnerabilities and their inability to achieve everything, they are free to make warm and ordinary relationships with their patients, family, and friends. They are free to look at the quality of their work and to make changes where these are needed. *The losses are losses of illusions; the gains are gains in reality,* and the quality of work and the quality of life can improve beyond recognition.

Further reading

Bennet G. *The wound and the doctor: healing, technology and power in modern medicine.* London: Secker and Warburg, 1987.

14 Assumptions about loss and principles of care

COLIN MURRAY PARKES

In this book we have examined the psychological consequences of the many losses that are encountered by members of the caring professions in the course of their work and considered the implications of these for the care of patients, their families, and ourselves. The defining characteristic of a loss is the grief to which it gives rise and the defining characteristic of grief, without which it cannot truly be said to be present, is pining, the feeling of missing the lost person, thing, situation, or other object to which one has been attached. This is evident in situations as varied as the amputee's yearning to run and jump (p 47), the separated partner's pining for a former wife or child (p 39), the blind person's need to continue to watch television in preference to listening to the radio (p 61), or the unemployed person's longing for a job, the workmates he or she has lost, and the self image that came with these (p 74).

Given this common ground we shall recapitulate by attempting to draw out *the assumptions that it is reasonable to make* in our current state of knowledge about the losses met with in medical practice and deduce from these *the principles of care that follow*. This approach has been used by the members of the *International Work Group on Death, Dying and Bereavement* as a means of reviewing current knowledge of the field and making recommendations.[1] It combines a clear statement of current assumptions in a refutable form with a linked statement of the principles that follow, also in a refutable form. Hence it should stimulate further research as well as providing guidelines for action.

Box 14.1 Summary of assumptions about loss and principles of care

Assumptions

Principles of care

- Major losses are important experiences that can contribute to causing physical and psychiatric illness

Members of the caring professions need to learn how to reduce the risk

- Losses that have been expected and prepared for are much less likely to give rise to later psychiatric and other problems than losses that are unexpected

By sensitively imparting information and support we can help people to prepare for the losses that are to come

- Many of the losses that are met within medicine affect the lives of members of the families of our patients

It is the family, which includes the patient, that should be the unit of care

- Grieving people tend to oscillate between avoiding and confronting grief, problems arise when either of these ways of coping predomiantes

Some people need permission and encouragement to grieve and reassurance of the normality of grieving

People may also need permission and reassurance that they do not have to grieve all of the time. They may need opportunities and encouragement to replan their lives in a way that values the past

- Anger and shame can complicate the course of grief

We need to reserve judgment and show understanding

- The minority at special risk can be identified before or at the time of a loss. These include those with traumatic losses, personal vulnerability, and lack of social support

Members of the caring professions are well placed to assess risk, to give support, and to advise those who need additional help how to get it

- Losses can affect the carer as well as the cared for. Doctors are not immune to grief

We need to become aware of our own reactions to our patients and their illnesses and to acknowledge and seek to meet our own needs for support

Contribution to other illness

A basic assumption that emerged repeatedly in the course of the book is the recognition that *major losses are important experiences that can contribute to causing physical and psychiatric illness.* Evidence to support this view was given in several chapters and the assumption would seem to be uncontroversial. The principle that follows from it is that *members of the caring professions need to take steps to acquaint themselves with the losses that afflict their patients.* Sadly we often fail to do this, either because we do not take steps to find out how our patients and their families are affected by the life events that are impinging on them or because, knowing the facts of the loss, we fail to discuss them because we are reluctant to upset or be upset by the patient. Thus, as reported in the preceding chapters, neither women undergoing mastectomy (p 50), mothers having a baby (p 86), or people in residential care who had suffered a bereavement (p 83) were encouraged to talk about the experience or asked how it will affect their lives.

Of course there would be no point in discussing these issues unless there was something that we could do to reduce the harmful effects of psychological trauma. Fortunately there are good grounds to believe that appropriate intervention can often reduce that risk (see, for example, p 26 & p 34). It follows from this that members of the caring professions need to ensure that such help is given when it is needed. This makes it important for us to ensure that doctors are trained to assess risk and take appropriate action.

Be prepared

Research into risk factors justifies the assumption that *losses that have been anticipated and prepared for are much less likely to give rise to later psychiatric and other problems than losses that are unexpected.* This has been shown to be true in regard to bereavement (p 15), operative surgery (p 52), and terminal care (p 103). The principle that follows is that *by sensitively imparting information and support we can help people to prepare for the losses that are to come.* Members of the caring professions are often in a position to do this but may fail to do so. Thus children are seldom warned of the likely death of a seriously ill parent (p 32) and surgical patients may be inadequately prepared for the consequences of the surgery. When anticipatory guidance has been given, however, the results are usually good (see p 52).

Many of the losses that are met with in medicine affect the lives of members of the families of our patients, and sometimes their losses are as great as or greater than those experienced by the patient. For instance, patients with Alzheimer's disease or other psychotic illnesses may be blissfully unaware that they are ill at all while their close relatives may be suffering severe grief (p 68 and pp 84–5). *Whenever a loss extends to affect the family it is the family, which includes the patient, that should be the unit of care.* This conclusion may seem obvious but members of the medical profession are so used to treating the patient as the unit of care that we regularly neglect the family. Thus, one study showed that 11 out of 12 families of psychiatric patients who had committed suicide would have liked some contact with the psychiatrist who had cared for the person who died but only one psychiatrist had initiated any such contact.[2] Even the simple process of recording who is who in the family by drawing a genogram (family tree) in the case notes is seldom done. A genogram displayed on a flip chart during case conferences and other meetings at which family needs are being considered is an effective way of helping the team to focus on family problems. In general practice, where it is common for doctors to get to know entire families over many years, genograms have proved particularly helpful (see Markus, *et al*[3] for a more detailed account of their use).

Pendulum of grief

While grieving people tend to oscillate between avoiding and confronting grief, problems arise when either of these ways of coping predominates. Sometimes a decision to cope in a particular way arises out of the special circumstances of the situation. Thus a woman may feel unable to express her grief at becoming pregnant because she thinks that others will disapprove or a man may pretend that he is not upset by a diagnosis of cancer because he does not wish to be seen as a "wimp" (other examples of this type of problem were given in chapter 8). Conversely a widow may feel she owes it to her dead husband to grieve for him for ever. In other cases the tendency to avoid or express grief reflects a lasting personality trait as in the "avoiders" and "sensitisers" which have been referred to in several chapters (see pp 7–8 & p 53). After major losses either type may suffer pathological forms of grief or become depressed.

The danger of these types of problem can be minimised by appropriate action. Thus some people need permission and encouragement to grieve and members of the caring professions may be the only people in a position to give these. Our professional and confidential relationship may cause people to confide in us information that is known to few if any others.

People may also need permission and encouragement to stop grieving and reassurance that nobody needs to grieve all of the time. Grief is not a duty to the dead or a sign of virtue. Obsessive grief can sometimes become an excuse to avoid the dangers of confronting a potentially hostile world. Thus, it is easy to see why some people who have suffered a psychotic illness will shut themselves up at home and resist attempts at rehabilitation. If we blame or browbeat them we shall only increase their feelings of insecurity and fear.

Those who overreact to loss will benefit from opportunities to re-examine their negative assumptions about themselves and their world, to review and replan their lives in ways that value and build on the past, and to venture forth into a world that seems more dangerous than it really is. Nothing succeeds like success and quite small beginnings can lead to a restoration of confidence that eventually allows great progress to be achieved. There is much to be said for John Bowlby's claim that "*the most important thing that we have to offer frightened or grieving people is a 'secure base'*",[4] a relationship of respect that will last them through the bad times with a person who has the time, knowledge, and willingness to remain involved.

Complicated grief

Feelings of *anger and shame can complicate the course of grief.* For example, mental illnesses or sexually transmitted diseases carry so severe a stigma that patients and relatives often fear that they will lose the support of friends and family if they acknowledge its existence let alone seek help or support for themselves. This adds to any stress that may have caused the illness. We need to reserve judgment and show understanding if we are to create the situation in which they can face up to what has happened and talk through its implications.

While most people come through the losses in their lives without the need for help from outside the family there is a minority who need such help. *The minority at special risk can be identified before or at the time of a loss.* This has been demonstrated in several studies (see p 15 and pp 76–7). The recognition of these risk factors enables us to give extra help when it is most needed and to conserve our resources when it is not. It follows that *members of the caring professions are well placed to assess risk,* to give support, and to advise those who need additional help how to get it.

Risk factors include traumatic losses, personal vulnerability, and lack of social support. Traumatic losses were considered in chapter 12. They include disasters and other situations in which losses are sudden, unexpected, horrific, or culpable. Ill health often adds to vulnerability and may itself bring people into our care. We need to cultivate sensitivity to the possible psychological influences of the physical illnesses that come our way.

Other causes of vulnerability are childhood and old age. Each carries with it particular hazards which need to be understood if we are to give appropriate help. Children were given special consideration in chapters 3 and 11 and elderly people in chapter 9. The hazards of losses in childhood often result from misguided attempts to protect a child, as when a parent conceals important information from a child or fails to seek psychiatric help for a child with learning difficulties. In old age it is more often the false assumption that losses are inevitable and that there is nothing to be done that deters old people from seeking help and care givers from offering it. Clinical depression often remains untreated and loneliness is assumed to be inevitable. Thus situations that may have been caused by loss result in further losses.

Sometimes the expectation of a loss can bring about a loss. A woman who has had a bad experience of pregnancy may experience high levels of anxiety and a propensity to depression which may spoil her next pregnancy. Similarly we saw on pp 51–2 how fear of further damage to the heart can impair the rehabilitation of heart surgical patients and, on page 63, how an overprotective spouse can impair the recovery of a blind person. In such circumstances medical and nursing professionals may need to give extra support and reassurance.

We saw in chapter 6 how *losses which impair communication disable the care giver as well as the cared for.* This makes it hard for us to support them if they are grieving or afraid. Above all we should take care not to allow our own feelings of irritation with the situation to spoil our relationship with our patients. It is not their fault that their behaviour is difficult.

Don't forget the care givers

In this, as in other clinical situations, we need to be aware of how our work is affecting us. As we saw in chapter 13, losses can affect the carer as well as the cared for and *doctors are not immune to grief.* The obstetrician who witnesses the death of a pregnant woman, the psychiatrist whose depressed patient commits suicide, and the general practitioner who has to break the news that a person whose backache has been misdiagnosed has an inoperable cancer are bound to be distressed.

We need to become aware of our own reactions to our patients and their illnesses and to acknowledge and seek to meet our own needs for support. In fact losses of one sort or another are so common in the lives of most doctors that it is good practice to hold regular meetings with a trusted group of colleagues at which we can support each other. If we do this we will come through the process of grieving and be able to return to the fray with renewed confidence. The very process of sharing genuine feelings with colleagues can help the group to cohere and leave us feeling more rather than less secure. We are no longer alone.

It is both the privilege and the penalty of being a part of a health care team that we will meet people who are suffering in the face of loss. If we back off or fail to recognise their needs we may miss the opportunity to help them through a turning point in their lives. We may also miss the opportunity to learn from them that *losses are often integrating factors in family life and, in the end, a source of new meaning and maturity.*

1 Corr CA, Morgan JD, Wass H *Statements on death, dying and bereavement.* King's College, London: International Work Group on Death, Dying and Bereavement, 1993.

2 Brownstein M. Contacting the family after a suicide. *Canadian J Psychiatry* 1992; 37:208–12.
3 Markus AC, Parkes CM, Tomson P *et al*. *Psychological problems in general practice*. Oxford: Oxford University Press, 1989.
4 Bowlby J. *A secure base: clinical applications of attachment theory*. London: Routledge, 1988.

Appendix A:

Organisations in the United Kingdom providing training, advice or counselling to patients, their families and professional caregivers

Bereavement

The Compassionate Friends (for bereaved parents)
53 North Street, Bedminster, Bristol BS3 1EN. Tel. 0117 953
9639. Fax. 0117 966 5202

The Cot Death Helpline (24 Hour)   Tel. 0171 235 1721

Cruse Bereavement Care   126 Sheen Road, Richmond,
Surrey TW9 1UR. Tel. 0181 940 4818. Fax. 0181 940 7638.
Bereavement Helpline 0181 332 7227 (Monday–Friday
9.30am–5pm). Youth Line 0181 940 3131 (Friday 5–9pm,
Saturday 11am–6pm)

Foundation for the Study of Infant Deaths (FSIDS)
14 Halkin Street, London SW1 X7DP. Tel. 0171 235 0965

The Lesbian and Gay Bereavement Project   Vaughan M.
Williams Centre, Colindale Hospital, London NW9 5HG. Tel.
0181 455 8894. Fax. 0181 905 9250 (7am–12pm)

The Miscarriages Association   Tel. 01924 200799

The National Association of Bereavement Services
20 Norton Folgate, London E1 6DB. Tel./Fax. 0171 247 0617.
Referrals 0171 247 1080

Stillbirth And Neonatal Death Society (SANDS)
28 Portland Place, London W1N 4DE. Tel. 0171 436 7940

Winston's Wish (provides training for counsellors and local support for bereaved children)   c/o Palliative Care Team, Gloucestershire Royal Hospital, Great Western Road, Gloucester GL1 3NN. Tel. (01452) 394377. Fax. (01452) 394195

Relationship Problems

National Family Mediation   Tel. 0171 383 5993

Relate   Herbert Gray College, Little Church Street, Rugby CV21 3AP. Tel. 01788 573 241. Fax. 01788 535 007. Email relate@ukonline.co.uk

Disability and chronic illness

BACUP (Information and support on cancer by trained nurses)   3 Bath Place (off Rivington Street), London EC2A 3JR. Tel. 0171 613 2121

Breast Care and Mastectomy Association   15–19 Britten Street, London SW3 3TZ. Tel. 0171 867 1103 (10am–5pm)

British Colostomy Association   15 Station Road, Reading, Berks RG1 1LG. Tel. 0118 939 1537

Cancerlink (Resource for cancer patients)   11–21 North Down Street, London N1 9BN. Tel. 0171 833 2451. Fax. 0171 833 4963

Carer's National Association   1 Castle Mews, Castle Road, North Finchley N12 9EH. Tel. 0181 343 9698

DIAL-UK   The Disability Helpline Tel. 01302 310123

Disabled Living Foundation   380–384 Harrow Road, London W9 2HU. Tel. 0171 289 6111

Hysterectomy Support   c/o Women's Health 52 Featherstone Street, London EC1Y 8RT. Tel. 0171 251 6580

Hodgkins Disease Association   PO Box 275 Haddenham, Aylesbury, Bucks. HP17 8JJ. Tel. 0184 429 1500

Issue The National Fertility Association   114, Lichfield Street, Walsall WS1 2SZ. Tel. 01922 722 888

Let's Face It (for those with facial disfigurement)   10 Wood End, Crowthorne, Berks. RG11 6DQ Tel. 0134 477 4405

Limbless Association   Rehabilition Centre Roehampton Lane, London SW15 5PR. Tel. 0181 788 1777. Fax. 0181 788 1777

The London Lighthouse (Support to those with problems relating to HIV infection)   111–117 Lancaster Road, London W11 1QT. Tel. 0171 792 1200

MIND (National Association for Mental Health)   Head Office Granta House 15–19 Broadway, Stratford, London E15 4BQ. Tel. 0181 519 2122

National AIDS Helpline (24 hour. Call free)   Tel. 0800 567123

National Association of Laryngectomy Clubs   Ground Floor, 6 Rickett Street, Fulham, London SW6 1RU Tel. 0171 381 9993. Fax. 0171 381 0025

Oesophageal Patient's Association   16 Whitefields Crescent, Solihull, West Midlands B91 3NY. Tel. 0121 704 9860

RADAR (The Royal Association for Disability and Rehabilitation)   Tel. 0171 250 3222

Terence Higgins Trust Helpline (AIDS)   Tel. 0171 242 1010

Urostomy Association   Buckland Beaumont Park, Danbury, Essex CM3 4DE
Tel. 01245 224294

Sensory and cognitive disorders

Alzheimer's Disease Society   Bedford Hall Bedford Road.
London W13 0PS. Tel. 0181 579 0079

The Association of Blind Asians   322 Upper Street, London
N1 2XO. Tel. 0171 388 2555

Carer's National Association (for relatives and others
providing care)   1 Castle Mews, Castle Road, North Finchley
N12 9EH. Tel. 0181 343 9668

Hearing Concern   7–11 Armstrong Road, London W3 7JL.
Tel. 0181 743 1110 or 0181 742 9151

MENCAP   for families affected by learning difficulties. Tel.
0171 454 0454

The Royal National Institute for the Blind (RNIB)
(Customer Services)   PO Box 173, Peterborough PE2 JWS.
Tel. 0345 023 153

The Royal National Institute for Deaf People
19–23 Featherstone Street, London EC1Y 8SL.
Tel. 0171 296 8000

Infertility and childbirth

National Childbirth Trust   National Headquarters Alexandra
House, Oldham Terrace, London W3 6NH. Tel. 0181 992 8637
(9.30am–4.30pm)

Old age

Age Concern   Astral House 1268 London Road, London
SW16. Tel. 0181 679 8000

Alzheimer's Disease Society   223 Windmill Road, London
W5. Tel. 0181 579 0079

Carer's National Association 1 Castle Mews, Castle Road, North Finchley N12 9EH. Tel. 0181 343 9698

Terminal illness

European Association for Palliative Care National Cancer Institute Milan, Via Venezian, 1 20133 Milan, Italy. Tel. 00392 2390792. Fax. 00392 70600462

Help the Hospices 34–44 Britannia Street, London WC1X 9JG. Tel. 0171 278 5668

The Hospice Information Service St Christopher's Hospice, 51–59 Lawrie Park Road, London SE26 6DZ. Tel. 0181 778 9252 ext. 262–263. Fax. 0181 776 9345

National Hospice Organization 1901 North Moore Street, Suite 901, Arlington, Virginia 22209, USA. Tel. 001203 7671620

Traumatic stress and disasters

For advice:
Disaster Planning and Limitation Unit Dept of Industrial Technology University of Bradford, Bradford, West Yorkshire BD7 1DP. Tel. 01274 733 466 ext. 8419

European Society for Traumatic Stress Studies Traumatic Stress Clinic, 73 Charlotte Street, London WIP 1LB. Tel. 0171 530 3666.

For adults and children affected by trauma:
Traumatic Stress Clinic (A national referral and training centre for adults, children and families) 73 Charlotte Street, London W1P 1LB. Tel. 0171 530 3666.

Rape Crisis Centre Tel. 0171 837 1600

Support after Murder or Manslaughter 39 Brixton Road, London SW9 6DZ. Tel. 0171 735 3838. Fax. 0171 735 3900

For library and computer database:
Office of the United Nations Disaster Relief Coordinator
(UNDRO) Palais des Nations, CH-1211 Geneva 10,
Switzerland. Tel. 34 60 11

For training in disaster management:
Centre for Crisis Psychology Pinetum Broughton Hall,
Skipton, North Yorks BD23 3AE. Tel. 01756 796383

**Crisis Training and Educational Counselling
(CRITEC)** Accident and Emergency Department, Leeds
General Infirmary, Great George Street, Leeds LS1 3EX. Tel.
0113 292 6498

Emergency Planning College The Hawkhills, Easingwold,
York YO6 3EG. Tel. 01347 821406

Support to doctors

BMA Stress Counselling Service Tel. 0645 200169

Appendix B:

Organisations in the United States providing training, advice or counselling to patients, their families and professional caregivers

Bereavement

Amend (Aiding Mothers and Fathers following Neonatal Death) One-to-one peer counselling with trained volunteers.
AMEND, 4324 Berrywick Terrace, St Louis, MO 63128
Tel. (001) (314) 487 7582

American Association of Suicidology (For survivors of suicide) Self-help groups for survivors of suicide nationwide. Newsletter, pamphlets etc.
American Association of Suicidology, 4201 Connecticut Ave., NW, #310, Washington, DC 20008. Tel. (001) (202) 237 2280

Association for Death Education and Counseling (For all concerned with dying, death and bereavement) Education, conferences, newsletter, accreditation of death educators, grief counsellors and grief therapists, code of ethics, advocacy, referrals and special interest groups.
ADEC, 638 Prospect Avenue, Hartford, CT 06105-4250
Online contact: http://www/adec.org/index.htm

The Beginning Experience (For divorced, windowed and separated adults and their children) Support groups.
The Beginning Experience, 1209 Washington Blvd., Detroit, MI 48226. Tel. (001) (313) 965 5110 Fax (001) (313) 965 5557

The Compassionate Friends (For parents and siblings grieving the death of a child) Support, friendship and

understanding. Telephone support, monthly chapter meetings, information, newsletter and resource guide.
The Compassionate Friends, PO Box 3696, Oak Brook, IL 65022. Tel. (001) (630) 990 0010 Fax (001) (630) 990 0246. Online contact: http://www.compassionatefriends.org

Parents of Murdered Children (For persons who survive the violent death of someone close) Self-help groups, newsletter and, in many areas, court accompaniment.
Parents of Murdered Children, 100 E 8th Street, B-41, Cincinnati, OH 45202. Tel. (001) (513) 721 5683 Fax (001) (513) 345 4489
Online contact: mailto:Nat1POMC@aol.com

Rainbows (For children or adults who are grieving death, divorce or other painful transition) Peer support groups led by trained adults. Newsletter, information and referrals.
RAINBOWS, 1111 Tower Rd., Schaumburg, IL 60173. Tel. 800 266 3206 or (001) (847) 310 1880 Fax (001) (847) 310 0120
Online contact: http://www.rainbows.org

Share: Pregnancy and Infant Loss Support, Inc. (For bereaved parents and families who have suffered miscarriage, stillbirth or neonatal death) Mutual support, newsletter, pen pals, information etc.
SHARE, c/o St. Joseph's Health Ctr., 300 First Capital Dr., St. Charles, MO 63301-2893. Tel. 800 821 6819 or (001) (314) 947 6164 Fax (001) (314) 947 7486
Online contact: http://www/nationalshareoffice.com

SIDS Alliance (For families of sudden infant death syndrome victims) Emotional support through local chapters. Supports research, educates the public. Newsletter and telephone support network.
SIDS Alliance, 1314 Bedford Ave., #210, Baltimore, MD 21208. Tel. (001) 800 221 7437, or, within Maryland (410) 653 8226 Fax (001) (410) 653 8709

THEOS (They Help Each Other Spiritually) (For widowed persons and their families) Mutual self-help in local groups.

THEOS, 322 Boulevard of the Allies, #105, Pittsburg, PA 15222-1919. Tel. (001) (412) 471 7779 Fax (001) (412) 471 7782

Unite, Inc. (For parents, grieving miscarriage, stillbirth and infant death) Group meetings, phone help, support for parents through subsequent pregnancies, newsletter, annual conference. Group facilitator and counsellor training programmes. Professionals in advisory roles.
Unite, Inc., Janis Heil, Jeannes Hospital, 7600 Central Ave., Philadelphia, PA 19111 2499. Tel. (001) (215) 728 3777 (tape) or (001) (215) 728 4286

Widowed Persons Service (For widows and widowers) One-to-one peer support, support groups, newsletter and referral services.
WPS, 601 E Street NW, Washington DC 20049.
Tel. (001) (202) 434 2260 Fax (001) (202) 434 6474
Online contact: mailto:astudner@aarp.org or http://www/aarp.org

See also below **Parents without Partners**

Relationship problems

See also above **The Beginning Experience** and **Rainbows**

CODAS (Children of Divorce and Separation). Consultation in areas of child custody, visitation, child support and guardian ad litem services.
Dr. Ken Lewis, CODAS, PO Box 202, Glenside, PA 19038.
Tel. (001) (215) 576 0177 Fax: (001) 576 9411.
Online contact: http://www/inc/com/users.CODAS.html

Divorce Care (For people in separation and divorce) Network of support groups, information and referral.
Divorce Care, 223 S. Whitem PO Box 1739, Wake Forest, NC 27587. Tel. (001) (919) 562 2112 Fax (001) (919) 562 2114
Online contact: http://www.divorcecare.com

Joint Custody Association (For divorcing parents who wish to achieve joint custody). Information re. family law, research and judicial decisions. Advocates legislative improvements.
c/o James A. Cook, 10606 Wilkins Ave., Los Angeles, CA 90024.
Tel. (001) (310) 475 5352

National Association for Fathers (For fathers and grandparents in divorce situations). Mutual support and advocacy, information, referrals, telephone support, conferences and literature.
National Association for Fathers, PO Box 877, Saylorsburg, PA 18353. Tel. 800 HELP DAD Fax (001) (717) 992 9380

Parents Without Partners (For single parents – divorced, separated, widowed or never married) Mutual help in local chapters, newsletter etc.
PWP, 401 N. Michigan Ave. Chicago, IL 60611-4267. Tel. 800 637 7974 or (001) (312) 644 6610 Fax (001) (312) 5144

Disablement and chronic illness

See also above, **Association for Death Education and Counseling**

American Amputee Foundation, Inc. Information, referrals and peer support for amputees. Hospital visitation and counselling, magazine, national resource directory for patients, families and caregivers. 'Give a Limb' programme.
American Amputee Foundation, Inc, PO Box 250218, Little Rock, AR 72225-0218. Tel. (001) (501) 666 2523 Fax (001) (501) 666 8367

American Cancer Society Provides research and patient services including information about cancer, public education, transportation, lodgings, children's camps etc. See also **Candlelighters** and **Man to Man Program**
Tel. 800 ACS 2345
Online contact: http://www.cancer.org

Amputee Coalition of America. (For amputees, professionals and disability-related organisations) Coalition of organisations

148

established to provide outreach, education and empowerment for amputees. Referrals to support groups.
Amputee Coalition of America, PO Box 2528, Knoxville, TN 37901-2528. Tel. 800 355 8772 Fax (001) (423) 525 7917
Online contact: mailto:ACAOne@aol.com

Candlelighters Childhood Cancer Foundation (For parents of children and adolescents with cancer, health and educational professionals) Links parents, families and groups to share feelings, exchange information, identify patient and family needs. Newsletter, youth newsletter and educational materials.
Candlelighters Childhood Cancer Foundation, 7910 Woodmont Ave., Suite 460, Bethesda, MD 20814. Tel. 800 366 2223 or (001) (301) 657 8401.
Online contact: http://www.candlelighters.org

International Association of Laryngectomees Practical and emotional support starting before laryngectomy and through rehabilitation. Newsletter.
International Association of Laryngectomees, 7440 N. Shadeland Ave., Suite 100, Indianapolis, IN 46250. Tel. (001) (317) 570 4568 Fax (001) (317) 570 4570.

Make Today Count (For persons facing a life-threatening illness including relatives and friends) Mutual support and discussion through local chapters.
c/o St. John's Regional Health Center, Mid-America Cancer Center, 1235 E. Cherokee St., Springfield, MO 65804-2263. Tel. Connie Zimmerman 800 432 2273 (Mid-America Cancer Center) Fax (001) (417) 888 8761

Man to Man Program (For men with Prostate Cancer) Support group meetings, phone support, information, referrals, education, support visiting programme and newsletter.
Tel. American Cancer Society 800 ACS 2345
Online contact: http://www.cancer.org

Mended Hearts (For persons with heart disease, families and friends) Support groups through local chapters, magazine.
Mended Hearts, 7272 Greenville Ave., Dallas, TX 75231.
Tel. (001) (214) 706 1442 Fax (001) (214) 987 4334
Online contact: http://www.mendedhearts.org

National Limb Loss Information Center Information, advocacy and advice.
National Limb Loss Information Center, Amputee Coalition of America, 900 East Hill Avenue, Suite 285, Knoxville, TN 37915-2568. Tel. (001) (423) 524 8772 Fax (001) (423) 525 7917
Toll-free 1 (888) 267 5669
Online contact: http://www.amputee-coalition.org

Reach to Recovery (For persons with cancer) One-to-one visitation and, in some areas, support groups.
Tel. American Cancer Society 800 ACS 2345
Online contact: http://www.cancer.org

Y-ME National Breast Cancer Association (For breast cancer patients and their families during all stages of the illness) Community outreach, information and peer support, hotline, newsletter and conferences.
Y-Me, 212 W. Van Buren Street, Chicago, IL 60607-3908
Tel. 800 221 2141 (24 hours) Fax (001) (312) 986 0020
Online contact: http://www.y-me.org

United Ostomy Association (Persons with ostomies and related surgery) Support through local chapters, visitation programme, education, magazine, national identity and support groups for parents of children with ostomies.
United Ostomy Association, 19772 MacArthur Blvd., Suite 200, Irvine, CA 92612-2405. Tel. 800 826 0826 or (001) (714) 660 8624 Fax (001) (714) 660 9262
Online contact: http://www.uoa.org

Sensory, motor and cognitive disorders

Alzheimer's Disease and Related Disorders Assoc. Inc (for caregivers) Information and assistance through local support groups, newsletters and literature.
ADRDA, 919 N. Michigan Ave., Suite 1000, Chicago, IL 60611-1676. Tel. 800 272 3900 or (001) (312) 335 8700 TDD (001) (312) 335 8882
Online contact: http://www.alz.org

American Council for the Blind (For blind and visually impaired people and their families) Support groups, phone support, information, referrals, education, advocacy, magazine and national conference.
American Council of the Blind, 1155 15th St. NW, #720, Washington, DC 20005. Tel. 800 424 8666 or (001) (202) 467 5081 Fax (001) (202) 467 5085
Online contact: http://www.acb.org

The Lighthouse, Inc (For older adults with impaired vision) Information and directory of member-run self-help groups and professionally-run support groups, information on low-vision clinics, vision rehabilitation agencies, products, assistive technology and newsletter.
The Lighthouse, Inc., 111 E. 59th Street, New York, NY 10022 Tel. 800 334 5497 (Voice), (001) (212) 9713 (TTY) & (001) (212) 821 9200 (general).
Online contact: http://www.lighthouse.org

National Association of the Deaf Information, publications, advocacy, accreditation of professionals, legal assistance, research etc.
National Association of the Deaf, 814 Theyer Ave., Silver Spring, MD 20910-4500. Tel. (001) (301) 587 1789 (TTY) or (001) (301) 587 1788 Fax (001) (301) 789 1791

National Federation of the Blind Contacts newly blind people to help with adjustment, information, student scholarships, literature and magazine.
National Federation of the Blind, 1800 Johnson St., Baltimore, MD 21230. Tel. (001) (410) 659 9314 or 800 638 7518 (for blind people seeking employment)
Online contact: http://www.nfb.org

National Fraternal Society for the Deaf (For the deaf and hard of hearing, their families and concerned professionals) Self-help organisation.
National Fraternal Society of the Deaf, 1118 S. Sixth Street, Springfield, IL 62703
Tel. (001) (217) 789 7438 (TDD) or (001) (217) 789 7489
Online contact: mailto:104656.272@compuserve.com

National Stroke Association (For people who have experienced strokes, their families and friends) Guidance for starting Stroke Clubs and groups, newsletter, professional publication, information, research fellowships and referrals.
National Stroke Association, 96 Inverness Dr., East Suite 1, Englewood, CO 80112-5112. Tel. (001) (303) 649 9299 or 800-STROKES Fax (001) (303) 649 1328
Online contact: http://www.stroke.org

National Aphasia Association (For patients, families and general public) Educates public about aphasia, information, referrals to local groups, magazine, young people's network and parents' network.
National Aphasia Association, 156 Fifth Ave., Suite 707, New York, NY 10011. Tel. 800 922 4622
Online contact: http://www.aphasia.org

Stroke Clubs International (For people who have experienced strokes, their families and friends) Information and assistance to and about local Stroke Clubs and newsletter.
Stroke Clubs International, 805 12th Street, Galveston, TX 77550. Tel. (001) (409) 762 1022

Stroke Connection of the American Heart Association (For stroke survivors, their families and support groups) List of support groups, forum for stroke survivors and families, magazine, information, publications and referrals.
Stroke Connection, 7272 Greenville Ave., Dallas, TX 75231. Tel. 800 553 6321 (day) Fax (001) (214) 706 5231
Online contact: http://www.amhrt.org

Infertility, childbirth and parenting

Attachment Disorder Parents Nnetwork (For parents and professionals dealing with children with attachment disorders) Newsletter, phone support, information and referrals.
Attachment Disorder Parents Network, PO Box 18475, Boulder, CO 80308. Tel. (001) (303) 443 1446

Depression after Delivery (For women who have suffered post-partum depression) Telephone support, newsletter, pen pals, conferences and group development guidelines.
D.A.D., PO Box 1282, Morrisville, PA 19067. Tel. 800 944 4773 (leave name and address for info) or (001) (215) 295 3994
Online contact: http://www.beharenet.com/dadinc

NINE (National Infertility Network Exchange) Educational meetings, newsletter, talk line, library, advocacy and professional referral.
NINE, PO Box 204, East Meadow, NY 11554. Tel. (001) (516) 794 5772 Fax (001) (516) 794 0008
Online contact: mailto:NINE204@aol.com

No Kidding! (For married or single people who either have decided not to have children, are postponing parenthood, are undecided or unable to have children) Mutual support and social activities, group development guidelines and newsletter.
No Kidding! Box 27001, Vancouver, BC, Canada, V5R 6A8.
Tel. (001) (604) 538 7736 (24 hrs) Fax (001) (604) 538 7736
Online contact:
http://www.mypage.direct.ca/d/dsimmer/nokids.html

Resolve (For infertile couples and members of the public) Support groups and education for members of the public. Newsletter and publications.
Resolve, 1310 Broadway, Somerville, MA 02144-1731.
Tel. (001) (617) 623 0744 Fax (001) (617) 623 0252
Online contact: http://www.resolve.org

Mental and emotional problems

Mental Health Net Information and resource list for mental health.
Online contact: http://www.cmhc.com/

NAMI (National Alliance for the Mentally Ill) (For relatives and individuals affected by mental illness) Self-help groups, newsletters, anti-discrimination campaign, affiliate development guidelines.

NAMI, 200 N. Glebe Rd., #1015, Arlington, VA 22203-3754.
Tel. 800 950 6264 (for group referrals) or (001) (703) 524 7600
Fax (001) (703) 524 9094
Online contact: http://www.mani.org

The Relatives Project (For families and friends of those with mental and emotional problems) Self-help groups, assistance in starting new groups.
The Relatives Project, c/o Phyllis Berning, Abraham A. Low Institute, 550 Frontage Rd., #2797, Northfield, IL 60093.
Tel. (001) (847) 441 0445 Fax (001) (847) 441 0446

Terminal illness

The Hospice Information Service Provides information about and listing of hospices and other resources for terminally ill patients and their families throughout the world.
The Hospice Information Service, St Christopher's Hospice, 51–59 Lawrie Park Road, London SE26 6DZ, UK. Tel. 0181 778 9252 ext 262-263 Fax 0181 776 9345

National Hospice Organisation (For terminally ill, their families and professinal carers) Promotes quality care for the terminally ill by education and resources for patients and families. Information, professional interest networks, resource center and conferences.
National Hospice Foundation, 1901 North More Street, Suite 901, Arlington, VA 22209. Tel. (001) (703) 516 4928
Online contact: http://www.nho.org

Traumatic stress and disasters

The Disaster Center Resource for all concerned with disasters.
Online contact: http://www.disastercenter.com/agency.htm

National Voluntary Organisations Active in Disasters (VOAD) Coordinates planning, newsletter, education and outreach.
Online contact: http://www.nvoad@vita.org

United Nations Department of Humanitarian Affairs (DHA)
Coordination and emergency response.
United Nations Department of Humanitarian Affairs (DHA),
Palais des Nations-CH-1211 Geneva 10, Switzerland. Tel (+4122)
917 3290 3515 3512 Emergency only (+4122) 917 2010 Fax
(+4122) 917 0023 Telex 41 42 42 dha ch
Online contact: DHGVA@UN.ORG

Other sources of help

For information about a wide variety of self-help and other groups
for many different diseases and situations see:

American Self-Help Clearing House
Self-help source book, online
Online contact: http://www.cmhc.com/selfhelp/

Index

Printed in the United Kingdom
by Lightning Source UK Ltd.
2839